Gynecology and Obstetrics

Treatment Guidelines

Paul D. Chan, M.D.

Susan M. Johnson, M.D.

Current Clinical Strategies Publishing
PO Box 1753
Blue Jay, CA 92317
info@ccspublishing.com

Printed in USA
ISBN: 978-1-881528-30-2

Table of Contents

OBSTETRICS

Obstetrics Admission Evaluation

Admission Criteria for Normal Laboring Patients

Labor is characterized by cervical dilation of 3–4 cm or more with regular, painful contractions. Ruptured membranes are indicative of labor. Bloody show or complete cervical effacement with regular and painful contractions are characteristic of labor.

I.Preterm Labor
A. Preterm labor causes regular contractions before 37 weeks gestation with cervical dilation and effacement.
B.Preterm labor presents with contractions, cramping, pelvic pressure, spotting, and low back pain.
C. **Speculum Examination**
1. A speculum examination should always be done before digital examination.
2. The cervix should be examined for dilation, lesions, or bleeding.
3. A sample should be obtained from the posterior fornix with a swab for fetal fibronectin.
4. Collect sample from the lower vagina and rectum or perianal area for group B streptococcus culture.
5. Collect specimen for wet mount if vaginal infection is suspected.
6. Gonorrheaand chlamydia testing should be done if the patient is high risk or if no prenatal care.
D.**Cervical Examination**
1. Evaluate for cervical dilation by estimating the size of the internal os.
2. Multiparous women may have cervical dilation in the third trimester without other preterm labor.
3. If the patient has vaginal bleeding, perform ultrasound to exclude placenta previa before performing digital exam.
E. **Fetal Monitoring.** Evaluate fetal heart rate pattern and assess frequency of uterine contractions
F. **Ultrasound**
1. **A**bdominal ultrasound for fetal biometrics, amniotic fluid index, fetal presentation, and location of the placental.
2. Transvaginal ultrasound for cervical length
   a) Cervical length more than 30 mm indicates that preterm labor unlikely
   b) Cervical length 20–30 mm plus contractions indicates that preterm labor more likely
   c) Cervical length <20 mm plus contractions indicates high risk for preterm labor
G. **Laboratory Studies**
1.Urinalysis, urine culture, and urine drug screen
2.Prenatal labs
H. **Criteria for Preterm Labor Admission**
1. Persistent and painful contractions at a frequency of 6 or more per hour
2. Rupture of membranes
3. Vaginal bleeding
4. Dilation ≥3 cm and/or effacement ≥80%

I. **Fetal Fibronectin (fFN)**
1. Fetal fibronectin has a positive predictive value of less than 20%. Negative predictive value of 69–92%. A negative test excludes the occurance of preterm delivery in the next 1–2 weeks. A positive test is not predictive of preterm labor.
2. Fetal fibronectin testing is not reliable if the specimen is contaminated with blood, semen, or gel.
3. The fetal fibronectin test is not needed:
   a) Gestation <24 weeks or ≥34 weeks
   b) Membranes have ruptured
   c) Cervix is dilated more than 3 cm
   d) Intracervical exam or vaginal ultrasound in the last 24 hours
J. **Combination of Cervical Length and Fetal Fibronectin**
1. Collect fFN sample before vaginal ultrasound
2. If cervical length is greater than 30 mm, no fetal fibronectin testing is needed
3. If cervical length is 20 and 30 mm, perform fetal fibronectin testing

II. **Rupture of Membranes**
A. **Clinical Evaluation**
1. Rupture of membranes presents with a sudden vaginal gush of fluid.
2. Urinary incontinence is common in pregnancy.
3. Rupture of membranes is often associated with contractions or vaginal spotting due to cervical dilation and effacement.
B. **Speculum Examination**
1. Pooling of clear fluid in the vaginal vault indicates that rupture of membranes has occurred.
2. Assess for cervical dilation or vaginal bleeding. A group B streptococcus culture should be done. A drop of vaginal fluid should be smeared on a slide and allowed to dry (fern test).
C. **AmniSure Test** detects trace amounts of placental α-microglobulin-1 (PAMG-1, which is an amniotic fluid proteins. AmniSure has 97% positive agreement and 97% negative agreement with diagnosis by pooling and ferning. Speculum exam is not required for vaginal AmniSure collection.
D. **Digital Examination**
1. Intracervical digital exam is contraindicated if gestational age less than 34 weeks in patients with rupture of membranes because contractions may be stimulated and because of increased risk of infection.
2. If the pregnancy is 34 weeks or more and delivery is planned, cervical exam should be done to assess cervical status for induction of labor.
E. **Ultrasound**
1. The presence of decreased amniotic fluid volume suggests rupture of membranes.
2. Fetal biometry ultrasound should be performed if the mother has not had prenatal care.
F. **Disposition**
1. If rupture of membranes is confirmed, the mother should be admitted for labor induction if ≥34 weeks.
2. If workup is negative, fetal heart tone reassuring, and no preterm labor, the patient should be discharged.

Vaginal Bleeding

Common Causes of Vaginal Bleeding include labor, cervical lesions, infections, cervical trauma, placenta previa, and placental abruption.

I. **Clinical Evaluation**
   A. Gestational age should be assessed because vaginal bleeding in early pregnancy (i.e., <20 weeks) should be evaluated in the emergency department.
   B. Vaginal bleeding may result from trauma or intercourse.
   C. Previa, abruption, and trauma may cause sudden, significant vaginal bleeding
   D. Infections may cause chronic; slow bleeding of prolonged duration.
   E. Determine if vaginal bleeding is associated with contractions, low back pain, cramping, or leakage of amniotic fluid.
   F. Placenta abruption manifests with severe abdominal pain and uterine contractions.

II. **Physical Examination**
   A. Tachycardia and hypotension indicate severe bleeding.
   B. **Speculum exam:** Inspect the surface of the cervix, and determine if the bleeding originates from cervical os, external cervix, or vagina. If no bleeding is visible, perform fFN and wet smear.
   C. **Cervical exam:** A digital examination should be performed if no placenta previa is visible on ultrasound

II. **Laboratory Studies**
   A. If bleeding is significant, perform type and screen, INR, partial thromboplastin time, fibrinogen, and Kleihauer-Betke. If Rh is negative, give an injection of RhIG.

III. **Ultrasound**
   A. An ultrasound should be completed before vaginal exam to exclude placenta previa.
   B. Measure amniotic fluid index and determine the fetal presentation. Perform fetal biometry to assess gestational age
   C. **Fetal Monitoring:** A non-reassuring fetal heart tracing and frequent contractions indicate placenta abruption.

IV. **Disposition:** If placenta previa, placenta abruption, or labor is suspected, the mother should be admitted.

Hypertension

I. **Clinical Evaluation**
   A. Determine the gestational age of the fetus and determine if the patient has preexisting hypertension or new-onset hypertension.
   B. Symptoms of hypertension include persistent severe headache, abdominal pain in right upper quadrant or epigastrium, scotomata, visual changes, swelling of hands and face, decreased fetal movement, vaginal bleeding, and contractions

II. **Physical Examination**
   A. Blood pressure should be measured in the sitting position.
   B. Assess for leg edema.
   C. Perform cervical exam and calculate the Bishop score to determine readiness for induction of labor.

III. **Fetal Monitoring**: Assess fetal heart rate pattern

IV. **Laboratory Studies**
   A. Measure hematocrit, platelet, creatinine, AST, LDH, and uric acid
   B. Obtain a spot urine sample for urine protein-to-creatinine ratio, which correlates with 24h urine protein measurement

V. **Ultrasound**
   A. Assess amniotic fluid index and fetal biometry if no prenatal care.

VI. Assessment and Disposition

A. The criteria for preeclampsia is a systolic blood pressure ≥140 mmHg or diastolic ≥90 mmHg and ≥1+ protein or urine protein-to-creatinine ratio ≥0.4.

B. If the mother is ≥ 37 weeks, delivery is indicated.

Decreased Fetal Movement

I. Causes of Decreased Fetal Movement

A. Decreased fetal movement may indicate intrauterine fetal demise. Decreased fetal movements usually result from a fetal sleep cycles, which typically last for 60 min. Fetal movements may occur with maternal hypoglycemia. Hypoxia reduces fetal movements.

B. Fetal movement counting should be initiated at 28–32 weeks. Ten distinct fetal movements in two hours is reassuring.

C. Decreased fetal movement is assessed with a nonstress test and amniotic fluid index. If the NST and AFI are normal, the patient may be sent home. If the initial nonstress test is nonreactive, a vibroacoustic device should be used to stimulate the fetus.

D. Patients with oligohydramnios or persistent nonreactive nonstress testing should be admitted.

II. Fetal Movement Monitoring

A. The mother should lie on her left side with her hand on the stomach. Fetal movements should be counted daily in the evening for at least 1 hour. She should call if:

1. No fetal movement in 12 hours
2. Less than 3 movements in 1 hour or less than 10 movements in 2 hours of counting
3. Movements are half of the usual rate.

Trauma

I. Clinical Evaluation

A. Assess gestational age, use of seat belts, abdominal pain, vaginal bleeding, fetal movement, resuscitation, and trauma.

B. Perform ultrasound to evaluate fetal heart, presentation, placental location, gestation age, and amniotic fluid volume. Ultrasound will often miss placental abruption (low sensitivity).

C. Monitor fetal heart rate pattern contractions.

D. **Labs:** CBC, type and screen, INR, PTT, fibrinogen, Kleihauer-Betke stain, and urine drug screen.

E. Intrauterine fetal demise after trauma commonly results from placental abruption. Coagulopathy is common after intrauterine fetal demise and is treated with 4-6 units of packed red blood cells and fresh frozen plasma.

F. If the fetus is >16–20 gestational weeks, admit to labor and delivery.

II. Cesarean Delivery. Emergency cesarean delivery may be performed if maternal death is imminent or if the fetal heart rate pattern is nonreassuring.

III. Perimortem Cesarean

A. Perimortem cesarean section is indicated if the pregnancy is ≥24 week. The cesarean section should be done within 4 minutes of maternal cardiac arrest. Fetal survival is unlikely more than 15 min after maternal death.

B. Perimortem cesareansection uses a midline skin incision from for xiphoid to pubic symphysis. A classical uterine incision should be performed to deliver the fetus.

IV. Treatment of Trauma Patients in Labor

A. An ultrasound should assess biometry and amniotic fluid index.

B. If RhD negative or more if more than 30 ml of fetomaternal bleeding by Kleihauer-Betke stain, give 300 ug RhoGAM IM.

C. Continue fetal monitoring for at least 4 hours. If contractions are less than six per hour for four hours, abruption is unlikely.

D. Monitoring is indicated frequent contractions, nonreassuring FHT, vaginal bleeding, rupture of membranes, or severe trauma.

Labor and Delivery

Electronic Fetal Monitoring

Electronic fetal monitoring assesses fetal oxygenation status. The fetal brain controls the heart rate. Fetal heart monitoring will identify fetal brain hypoxia. Fetal heart monitoring has not been proven to decrease cerebral palsy or perinatal mortality.

I. Definitions

A. Baseline
1. The baseline rate is evaluated for at least 2 min. Fetal heart rate is rounded to increments of 5 bpm.
2. The normal baseline fetal heart rate is 110–160 beats per minute
3. Bradycardia is a baseline heart rate <110 bpm.
4. Tachycardia is a baseline heart rate >160 bpm.

B. Baseline Variability
1. Baseline variability is measured from peak to trough and excludes decelerations and accelerations.
2. Absent variability has an undetectable amplitude range
3. Minimal variability has an amplitude range ≤5 bpm
4. Moderate variability is 6–25 bpm
5. Marked variability is >25 bpm

C. Acceleration
1. An acceleration is an abrupt increase in fetal heart rate
2. At more than 32 weeks, variable decelerations are ≥15 bpm above baseline, and have a duration of more than 15 seconds.
3. At less than 32 weeks, variable decelerations are ≥10 bpm above baseline, and have a duration of more than 10 seconds.
4. A prolonged acceleration has a duration of 2 minutes to 10 min.
5. Accelerations can be elicited by scalp stimulation or vibroacoustic stimulation.

D. Decelerations
1. Variable Decelerations
a) Variable decerations are abrupt decreases in fetal heart rate with a decline of more than 15 bpm. Variable decelerations last ≥15 seconds to 2 minutes.
b) When associated with contractions, variable decelerations will have a variable onset, depth, and duration in relation to the contractions.
c) Variable decelerationsare the most common deceleration patterns and are usually caused by cord compression.

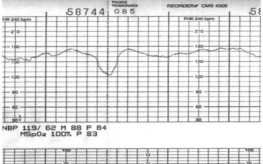

Figure: Variable decelerations

2. Late Decelerations

a) Late decelerations are symmetrical and have a gradual decrease
   and return to base line. Late decerations have an onset to nadir of
   ≥30 seconds and are associated with contractions. The onset and
   nadir of the late deceleration occurs after the peak of contractions.

b) Late decelerations are designated recurrent late decelerations if
   the decelerations occur with 50% or more of the contractions.

c) Intermittent late decelerations occur with <50% of contractions
   during a 20-minute period.

d) Late decelerations are caused by uteroplacental insufficiency.

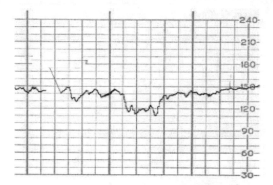

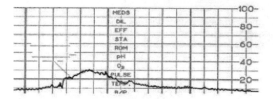

Figure: Late decelerations

3. **Early Decelerations**
   a) Early decelerations have a gradual decrease in fetal heart rate
      with onset to nadir ≥30 seconds. The early decelerations start with
      a contraction, and the nadir occurs simultaneously as the peak of
      the contraction.
   b) Early decelerations are caused by fetal head compression and
      are an infrequent pattern associated with active labor between 4–
      7 cm dilation.
   c) Early decelerations are not clinically significant, and labor may
      continue if early decelerations are present.

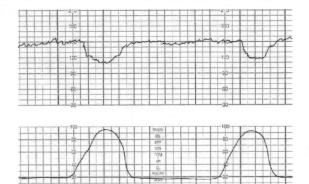

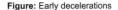

Figure: Early decelerations

E. Sinusoidal Fetal Heart Rate Pattern
  1. Sinusoidal fetal heart rate pattern has a sine wave-like undulating pattern with a cycle frequency of 3–5/min for more than 20 min.
  2. The sinusoidal pattern is infrequent but is associated with severe fetal anemia or acidosis

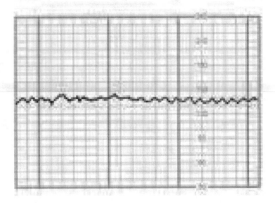

F. Prolonged Decelerations have a duration of more than 2 minutes, but are less than 10 minutes in duration.

G. Uterine Contractions
  1. Uterine contractions normally occur at a rate of 5 contractions in 10 minutes
  2. Tachysystole is more than 5 uterine contractions in 10 minutes and tachysystole is often associated with fetal heart rate decelerations.

5-Tier Fetal Heart Rate Classification

Category Green:

Normal baseline
Moderate variability
Early or mild Variable decelerations

Category Blue:

If moderate variability:
-Tachycardia with early or mild variable decelerations
-Normal baseline with moderate VD or mild late decelerations
If minimal variability:
-Tachycardia without decelerations
-Normal baseline ± early decelerations

Category Yellow:

If moderate variability:
-Tachycardia with moderate variable decelerations, mild/moderate late decelerations, or prolonged decelerations
-Normal baseline with severe VD, moderate/severe LD, mild/moderate prolonged decelerations
-Mild bradycardia ± early, mild/moderate VD, LD, or PD
-Moderate bradycardia ± early decelerations
If minimal variability:
-Tachycardia with early or mild VD
-Normal baseline with mild VD
Marked variability

Category Orange:

If moderate variability:
-Tachycardia with severe variable decelerations, LD, or Prolonged decelerations
-Normal baseline with severe Prolonged deceleration
-Mild bradycardia with severe VD, LD. or PD
-Moderate bradycardia with severe VD, LD, or PD
-Any severe bradycardia
If minimal variability:
-Tachycardia with moderate/severe VD, mild/moderate LD, or prolonged decelerations
-Normal baseline with moderate/severe VD, mild/moderate LD, or PD
-Mild or moderate bradycardia ± early deceleration
If absent variability:
-Normal baseline

Category Red

If minimal variability:
-Tachycardia with severe late decelerations
-Normal baseline with severe LD or PD
-Mild or moderate or severe bradycardia with any VD, LD, or prolonged decelerations
If absent variability:
-Any baseline with any deceleration
Sinusoidal

I. Interpretation of Fetal Heart Rate Tracings

A. Variable, late, or prolonged decelerations are signs of inadequate oxygen transfer to the fetus.

B. Moderate variability predicts absence of fetal metabolic acidemia.

C. Accelerations predict the absence of fetal acidemia.

D. Category Green Tracings
   1. **Acidemia:** None
   2. Actions: None

E. Category Blue Tracings
   1. **Acidemia:** Low risk of evolution
   2. Consider: Change to lateral position
   3. Give oxygen by mask
   4. Correct hypotension with a 500 mL normal saline IV bolus.
   5. Decrease oxytocin. Give terbutaline.
   6. Avoid constant pushing.
   7. Amnioinfusion if oligohydramnios
   8. Notify obstetrician
   9. Keep operating room available

B. Category Yellow Tracings
   1. **Acidemia:** None
   2. Moderate risk of deterioration
   3. Change to lateral position
   4. Oxygen
   5. Correct hypotension with 500 mL normal saline IV bolus
   6. Decrease oxytocin. Give terbutaline
   7. Amnioinfusion if oligohydramnios
   8. Obstetrician at bedside.
   9. Notify anesthesiologist and infant resuscitator and operating room available

C. Category Orange Tracings
   1. **Acidemia:** Potential for decompensation
   2. High risk of evolution
   3. Position change to lateral position
   4. Oxygen
   5. Correct hypotension with 500 mL normal saline IV bolus
   6. Stop oxytocin. Give terbutaline. Amnioinfusion if oligohydramnios.
   7. Prepare for urgent delivery
   8. Move patient to operating room
   9. Obstetrician and anesthesiologist should be present
   10. Infant resuscitator immediately available

D. Category Red Tracings
   1. **Acidemia:** Evidence of actual or impending fetal asphyxia
   2. Urgent delivery required
   3. Move patient to operating room
   4. Obstetrician, anesthesiologist, and infant resuscitator should be present

Management of Abnormal Fetal Heart Rate Patterns

I. **Ancillary Tests**
   A. Digital fetal scalp stimulation and vibroacoustic stimulation are frequently used to elicit fetal heart rate accelerations when category yellow or category orange tracings are present.

II. **Intrauterine Fetal Resuscitation**
   A. Reposition the mother in the left or right lateral position.
   B. Oxygen will raise the fetal umbilical arterial oxygen concentration.
   C. **Hydration:** An IV fluid bolus should be infused to correct hypotension. Ephedrine or phenylephrine should be given IV for hypotension due to regional anesthesia.
   D. Oxytocin should be stopped to relieve uterine tachysystoles. Tocolysis with terbutaline 0.25 mg IV or subcutaneous may be needed to stop contraction-induced decelerations.
   E. Examine the cervix and assess for cord prolapse. Perform an amniotomy. Place a fetal scalp electrode and insert an intrauterine pressure catheter. Recurrent variable decelerations should be treated with amnioinfusion.

III. **Treatment of Tachysystole**
   A. Tachysystole during spontaneous labor requires no intervention in category green or blue tracings. Tocolytics may be used in category yellow, orange, or red tracings.
   B. Oxytocin should be stopped and tocolytics given for category yellow, orange, or red tracings.

IV. **Treatment of Fetal Tachycardia**: Evaluate and treat maternal infections, fever, placenta abruption, medications, and hyperthyroidism, which may cause fetal tachycardia.
   A. **Treatment of Fetal Bradycardia**: Evaluate for maternal hypothermia, sepsis, and fetal heart disease.

V. **Treatment of Minimal Fetal Heart Rate Variability**
   A. Common etiologies of decreased fetal heart rate include fetal sleep, narcotics, magnesium sulfate, and fetal acidemia.
   B. Fetal scalp stimulation or vibroacoustic stimulation should be used to increase variability.

VI. **Treatment of Prolonged Deceleration**
   A. Prolonged decelerations may be caused by epidural or spinal anesthesia, prolonged compression on umbilical cord, eclampsia, placenta abruption, or cord prolapse.
   B. If intrauterine resuscitation is not effective, operative vaginal delivery or cesarean section is indicated.

VII. **Treatment of Variable Deceleration**
   A. Intermittent variable decelerations are variable decelerations that occur with <50% of contractions. Intermittent variable decelerations may not need interventions.
   B. Recurrent variable decelerations are variable decelerations that occur with ≥50% of contractions. Deep decelerations and prolonged variable decelerations in the absence of variability or accelerations are associated with fetal acidemia.
   C. Amnioinfusion relieves cord compression caused by oligohydramnios and reduces the cesarean rate and improves cord pH.
   D. Amnioinfusion Procedure: a bolus infusion of 500 ml of normal saline is followed by a continuous infusion of normal saline at 1 ml per min

VIII. Treatment of Recurrent Late Deceleration
   A. General resuscitation measures should be initiated to improve placental perfusion.
   B. If late decelerations persist with minimal variability and no accelerations, delivery should be accomplished.

IX. Medication Effects on Fetal Heart Rate Patterns
   A. $MgSO_4$ reduces baseline variability and inhibits in accelerations.
   B. Morphine decreases the frequency of accelerations.
   C. Betamethasone decreases fetal heart rate variability. Betamethasone may cause a decrease in the biophysical profile for 24 to 48 hours.
   D. Butorphanol (Stadol) causes a transient sinusoidal fetal heart rate pattern.
   E. Nalbuphine (Nubain) causes decreased frequency of accelerations and decreased variability.
   F. Cocaine causes increased contractions.
   G. Terbutaline decreases the frequency of late and variable decelerations.
   H. β-blockers may reduce the fetal heart rate.

X. Analgesia and Anesthesia
   A. **Parenteral Agents**
      1. Narcotics reduce fetal heart rate variability and reduce the Apgar score.
      2. Parenteral agents provide limited pain relief in labor and cause nausea and vomiting.
      3. **Parenteral Agents for Labor Pain**
         a) Fentanyl: 50–100 μg IV q1h
         b) Nalbuphine (Nubain): 10 mg IV q3h
         c) Morphine: 2–5 mg IV or 10 mg IM q4h
   B. **Neuraxial Anesthesia**
      1. Injection of lidocaine, bupivacaine, ropivacaine, fentanyl, or morphine into the lumbar space provides pain relief for labor and delivery.
      2. **Complications of Epidural Anesthesia**
         a) Fetal heart rate decelerations are treated with 0.25 mg of terbutaline IV or IM to relieve uterine tachysystole. If hypotension develops, give 5–10 mg of ephedrine (α and β receptor agonist) or 50–100 μg of phenylephrine (α1 receptor agonist).
         b) Epidural anesthesia is associated with increased rate of operative vaginal delivery, fever, and pruritus. High spinal block is infrequent. Epidurals may rarely cause seizure and cardiac arrest.
         c) Postepidural headache is treated with bed rest and oral analgesics. A blood patch 20 ml of patient's blood may be injected into the epidural space.
   B. **Spinal Anesthesia** is a short-acting anesthetic method, which is useful for cesarean delivery and postpartum tubal ligation
   C. **General Anesthesia**
      1. General anesthesia is associated with increased risk of maternal mortality.
      2. Anesthetic gas crosses the placenta and results in neonatal CNS depression.
      3. Uterine relaxation due to halogenated agents increases uterine postpartum hemorrhage.

Normal Labor and Delivery

I. **Mechanisms of Labor**
   A. **Power**
      1. The external tocometer monitors the frequency of contractions. External tocometers do not measure the strength of contractions.
      2. An intrauterine pressure catheter can monitor the pressure inside the uterus.
   B. **Passage**
      1. Clinical Pelvimetry. Clinical examination evaluates the pelvic shape and dimension. A trial of labor is the only reliable method of assessing the adequacy of birth passage.
   C. **Passenger**
      1. **Fetal Size.** Macrosomia is a fetal weight ≥4,500 grams. Macrosomia may result in failed labor. Clinical examination and ultrasound are not accurate in estimating fetal weight, especially at term.

II. **Pelvic Stations**
   A. 0 station is the level of ischial spines.
   B. At station +5, the head is visible at the introitus.

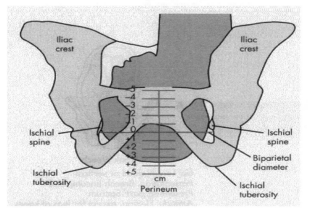

Figure: Pelvic stations

III. **Cardinal Movements of Labor:**
   A. Engagement is the first movement of labor
   B. Descent is the second movement, which occurs early in nulliparas.
   C. Flexion of the fetal head onto the chest presents the smallest presenting part.
   D. **Internal Rotation:** The fetus usually rotates from occiput transverse to left occiput anterior.
   E. Extension occurs at the introitus when the occiput extends under the symphysis.
   F. Restitution (external rotation) occurs when the head rotates from occiput anterior to left occiput transverse or right occiput transverse at perineum after delivery.
   G. Expulsion is delivery of anterior shoulder followed by posterior shoulder.

II. Stages of Labor

A. First Stage of Labor

1. The first stage of labor starts at the onset of labor (painful contractions q3–5 min) and continues until complete cervical dilation

2. **Latent phase**
   a) The latent phase of the first stage starts at the onset of labor and ends at 4 cm of cervical dilation
   b) **Prolonged latent phase** is defined as more than 20 hours in nulliparous or more than 14 hours in multiparous

3. **Active phase**
   a) The active phase of the first stage of labor begins at 4 cm cervical dilation and ends at complete cervical dilation
   b) The active phase is normally 5 hours in nulliparous. The minimum active phase rate of cervical dilation is 1.2 cm/hour in nullipara and 1.5 cm in a multipara.
   c) **Protraction disorder** is defined as cervical change of less than 1.2 cm per hour for a nullipara and 1.5 am in a multipara.

B. Second Stage of Labor

1. The second stage of labor begins with complete cervical dilation and ends with the delivery of infant.

2. The second stage for nulliparas is less than 2 hours without epidural, and less than 3 hours with an epidural.

3. The second stage of labor for multiparas is less than 1 hour without epidural, and less than 2 hours with an epidural.

C. Third Stage of Labor

1. The third stage of labor is delivery of the placenta, which usually occurs within 30 minutes after delivery of the newborn.

2. Delivery of the placenta starts with signs of cord separation, such as cord lengthening and a gush of blood

3. IV oxytocin is given after delivery of the placenta to decrease postpartum hemorrhage.

D. Cervical Examinations

1. Wear sterile gloves and use an index finger and a middle finger to palpate cervical dilation, effacement, fetal station, cervical position (anterior, midposition, and posterior), and cervix consistency (hard, moderate, soft). A bishop score greater than 6 is predictive of successful induction of labor.

2. Cervical dilation is a measurement of the dilation of internal os (not dilation of the external os).

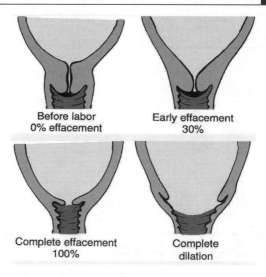

Before labor
0% effacement

Early effacement
30%

Complete effacement
100%

Complete
dilation

Figure: Cervical effacement

II. Management of Labor

A. Admit when cervix dilation is more than 3–4 cm or when active labor has started.

B. Sips of water and ice chips. Lactated ringers at 125 ml per hour IV

C. IV analgesics or epidural anesthesia

D. Oxytocin and artificial rupture of membranes are often given to augment labor (artificial rupture of membranes may be performed at cervix dilation >6–7 cm)

III. Labor Dystocia

A. Dystocia is slow and abnormal labor progression, which require cesarean section.

B. Labor augmentation is the use oxytocin and artificial rupture of membranes to stimulate uterine contractions.

IV. Arrest of Dilation in the First-Stage Labor

A. Cervical dilation of 4 cm or more

B. No cervical change for 2 hours with adequate contractions

V. Prolonged Second-Stage Labor

A. Prolonged second stage of labor may require operative delivery.

B. Labor may continue if the fetal heart tracing is reassuring.

C. Prolonged second stage of labor has a higher incidence of chorioamnionitis, third- or fourth-degree laceration, and uterine atony.

D. The management of persistent occiput posterior presentation is manual rotation to occiput anterior after complete cervical dilation.

VI. Labor Augmentation

A. High station, cervix <3 cm, not in active labor, malpresentation, and high HIV viral load.

B. Oxytocin

1. Oxytocin is produced in the hypothalamus and secreted by the posterior pituitary.

2. Maximum dose of oxytocin is 20 to 40 mU/min.

3. Oxytocin 10 or 20 units in 1 L of normal saline.

II. Management of Breech Presentation in Active Labor

A. Vaginal delivery of term breech is avoided due to neonatal morbidly and mortality.

B. Vaginal breech delivery may be allowed to proceed if a woman presents with frank breech and advanced cervical dilation or breech presentation of a second twin.

III. Meconium Staining of Amniotic Fluid

A. Meconium staining occurs in 12% deliveries, but is rare before 38 weeks

B. Meconium staining is associated with oligohydramnios and placental insufficiency.

C. Passing meconium is associated with neonatal meconium aspiration syndrome, low Apgar score, and cesarean delivery.

D. Intrapartum oropharyngeal and nasopharyngeal suction for meconium aspiration syndrome is indicated if the newborn has respiratory distress.

IV. Chorioamnionitis

A. Intraamniotic infection occurs in 2.0% of term pregnancies.

B. Chorioamnionitis is polymicrobial and pathogens include bacteroides, G. vaginalis, E. coli, group B streptococcus, and other gram negative-rods.

C. Risk factors for chorioamnionitis include prolonged labor, prolonged rupture of membranes, and internal monitors.

D. **Criteria for Diagnosis of Chorioamnionitis**

1. Maternal fever >38.0°C

2. Uterine tenderness, maternal tachycardia >110/min, fetal tachycardia >160/min, and foul amniotic fluid odor

3. WBC >15,000/mm3 with a left shift.

E. **Treatment**

1. Oxytocin is used to expedite delivery. Cesarean is performed for non-reassuring fetal heart tracings or dystocia.

2. Ampicillin 2 g q6h and gentamicin 1.5 mg/kg q8h (use clindamycin instead of ampicillin if β-lactam allergic). If cesarean is done, Metronidazole (Flagyl) 500 mg q12h is added.

3. Stop antibiotics after the patient afebrile for 24h postpartum.

Perineal Laceration and Episiotomy

I. Classification of Perineal Laceration

A. **First Degree Laceration** involves the fourchette, perineal skin, and vaginal mucosa

B. **Second Degree Laceration** involves the fascia and muscles of the perineal body

C. **Third Degree Laceration** involves the anal sphincter (partial or complete)

D. **Fourth Degree Laceration** extends through the rectal mucosa to expose the rectal lumen

II. Laceration Repair

A. **First-Degree Laceration.** First-degree perineal lacerations usually do not require repair.

B. **Second-Degree Laceration**

1. The second degree laceration is the most common type of laceration.

C. **Third-Degree Laceration**

1. If the anal sphincter is partially lacerated, reapproximate the lacerated sections with 2–0 interrupted sutures. The figure-8 suture should not be used because of muscle strangulation.

2. If the anal sphincter is completely lacerated, identify the cut end of the anal sphincter, and pull the sphincter together with Allis clamps. Reapproximate the muscle and capsule with 2–0 interrupted suture.

D. **Fourth-Degree Laceration**
   1. Incomplete repair of a forth-degree laceration may cause anal incontinence, and rectovaginal fistula.
   2. **Four–Layer Repair**
      a) Suture the rectal submucosa with running 4–0 Vicryl, 4–0 Monocryl, or 4–0 Chromic gut
      b) Reapproximate internal sphincter with running 4–0 Vicryl or 4–0 Monocryl.
      c) Reapproximate the external anal sphincter with 4 interrupted sutures.
      d) Repair the vaginal and perineal laceration.

Induction of Labor

I. **Indications for Induction of Labor**
   A. Fetal indications for induction include post-term pregnancy, rupture of membranes, chorioamnionitis, fetal demise, placenta abruption, severe intrauterine growth restriction, isoimmunization, and oligohydramnios
   B. Maternal indications for induction include preeclampsia, eclampsia, gestational hypertension, preexisting hypertension, diabetes, renal disease, pulmonary disease, and antiphospholipid syndrome
   C. **Criteria for Confirmation of Term Gestation**
      1. Ultrasound measurement at <20 weeks supports a gestational age of ≥39 weeks.
      2. Fetal heart tones have been documented t for 30 weeks by Doppler ultrasonography.
      3. 36 weeks have elapsed since a positive serum or urine human chorionic gonadotropin pregnancy test result.
   D. **Contraindications for Induction of Labor**
      1. Placenta previa or vasa previa
      2. Cord prolapse
      3. Malpresentation
      4. Previous classical cesarean or previous myomectomy entering the uterine cavity
      5. Active genital herpes

II. **Evaluation of Cervical Readiness for Induction**
   A. Simplified Bishop score includes: dilation, station and effacement. A simplified Bishop score >5 correlates with Bishop score of >8.

Bishop Score Evaluation of Cervical Readiness for Induction					
Scores	Dilation	Efface- ment	Station	Con- sistency	Position
0	Closed	0-30	-3	Firm	Posterior
1	1-2	40-50	-2	Medium	Midposition
2	3-4	60-70	-1,0	Soft	Anterior
3	≥5	≥80	+1, +2	-	-

III. **Cervical Ripening**
   A. Cervical ripening is indicated if the cervix is not favorable for induction of labor.
   B. **Mechanical Cervical Ripening**
      1. Intracervical Foley Catheter: Pass the balloon catheter just beyond the internal os, fill the balloon with 30 to 60 ml of normal saline, and apply traction on the catheter with a 500 to 1,000 mg weight.
   C. **Prostaglandins**
      1. Prostaglandins are contraindicated in woman with previous cesarean or other major uterine surgery.
      2. Misoprostol (Cytotec) is a synthetic prostaglandin E_1 analog
      3. 25 µg (1/4 of a 100 µg tab) placed in posterior fornix every 3–6 hours. Oxytocin is initiated 4 hours after the last dose of misoprostol.
      4. **Dinoprostone is a prostaglandin E_2 analog**
         a) Prepidil gel 0.5 mg, intracervical q6h, max 1.5 mg/24h. Start oxytocin 6–12 hours after the last dose of Prepidil.
         b) Cervidil 10 mg vaginal insert is a sustained release preparation, resolved over 12 hours. The insert can be easily removed. Oxytocin is started 30–60 minutes after removal of the insert.

Prolonged Pregnancy

I. Prolonged or post-term pregnancy is defined as a pregnancy of 42 weeks or more. 7% of pregnancies are prolonged. Erroneous dating is the most frequent cause of prolonged pregnancy.
   A. **Assessment of Gestational Age:** If there is a discrepancy between estimated date of delivery by LMP and the estimated date of delivery by ultrasound, the ultrasound estimate should be used.
   B. **Risks Associated with Post-term Pregnancy**
      1. Stillbirth and neonatal death
      2. Uteroplacental insufficiency, resulting in oligohydramnios, meconium aspiration, fetal distress in labor, low Apgar scores, and acidemia
      3. Macrosomia or growth restriction
      4. Increased cesarean delivery rate
II. **Treatment**
   A. Induction of labor at 41 weeks, regardless of cervical status is associated with a lower perinatal mortality.
   B. Deliver at 41 weeks if the cervix is favorable or if fetal compromise or oligohydramnios (amniotic fluid index <5).
   C. Antenatal testing should be initiated between 41 and 42 weeks with twice weekly amniotic fluid index and nonstress test.

Group B Streptococcal Prophylaxis

Group B streptococci colonize the rectum and vagina in 10% of pregnant women. Vertical transmission during labor can cause neonatal group B streptococcus sepsis, pneumonia, and meningitis.

I. **Universal Group B Streptococcus Screening**
   A. Screening for group B streptococcus is required for all patients at 35–37 weeks of gestation.
   B. Sample collection for group B streptococcus culture: Swab the lower vagina and rectum. A vaginal-perianal culture is an alternative.
   C. Group B streptococcus urinary tract infection should be treated with nitrofurantoin 100 mg q6h.

II. **Indications for Group B Streptococcus Prophylaxis**
   A. Invasive group B streptococcus disease with a previous infant
   B. Group B streptococcus bacteriuria (>10^4 cfu/ml) during the current pregnancy
   C. Positive group B streptococcus culture during the current pregnancy
   D. **Unknown group B streptococcus status at onset of labor and one or more of the following:**
      1. Less than 37 weeks
      2. Rupture of membranes for 18 hours or more
      3. Intrapartum fever ≥38.0°C or
      4. Intrapartum nucleic acid amplification test positive for group B streptococcus

III. **Nonindications for Intrapartum group B streptococcus Prophylaxis**
   A. Group B streptococcus colonization in previous pregnancy
   B. Group B streptococcus bacteriuria in previous pregnancy
   C. Negative group B streptococcus screening in late gestation during current pregnancy
   D. Cesarean before onset of labor with intact membranes, regardless of group B streptococcus status

IV. **Group B streptococcus Prophylaxis in Preterm Labor or Preterm-Premature Rupture of Membranes (< 37 Weeks)**
   A. Women with preterm labor or PPROM at admission, for group B streptococcus colonization should be screened unless it was done within the prior 5 weeks.
   B. Give group B streptococcus prophylaxis if the GBS unknown or if group B streptococcus status is positive.
   C. Antibiotics for group B streptococcus prophylaxis should be discontinued if the patient is not in true preterm labor or if group B streptococcus culture is negative.
   D. For patients with PPROM, group B streptococcus prophylaxis should be stopped at 48 hours if labor does not occur. Antibiotics that are given during the prolonged latency period are effective for group B streptococcus prophylaxis.
   E. A negative group B streptococcus screening culture is valid for 5 weeks. Repeat group B streptococcus screening is necessary if the culture was performed more than 5 weeks prior and patient is at risk of preterm delivery.

V. **Prophylactic Regimens**
   A. **No Allergy to Penicillin**
      1. One dose of penicillin G 5 million units IV for 1 then 2.5–3 million units IV q4h until delivery
      2. Alternative regimen: ampicillin 2g IV, then 1g IV q4h until delivery
   B. **Allergic to Penicillin**
      1. No history of anaphylaxis: cefazolin (Ancef) 2g IV for 1 then 1g IV every 4 hours until delivery
      2. History of anaphylaxis, angioedema, respiratory distress or urticaria: Give clindamycin 900 mg IV q8h until delivery if the GBS is susceptible to clindamycin and erythromycin.
         a) Test for inducible clindamycin resistance if group B streptococcus is susceptible to clindamycin but is resistant to erythromycin.
         b) Give vancomycin 1g IV q12h until delivery if group B streptococcus isolate is resistant to clindamycin.

VI. **Labor Management of Group B Streptococcus Positive Patient**
   A. Group B streptococcus prophylaxis is given for at least 4 hours before delivery. However, an obstetrical procedure should not be delayed to administer group B streptococcus prophylaxis.

Operative Vaginal Delivery

I. **Indications for Operative Vaginal Delivery by Vacuum or Forceps**
   A. Nonreassuring fetal heart rate pattern
   B. Prolonged second stage labor: nulliparas ≥2h without epidural, ≥3h with epidural. Multiparas ≥1h without epidural, ≥2h with epidural
   C. Maternal indications for operative vaginal delivery include exhaustion, insufficient expulsive efforts, or a medical reason to avoid maternal pushing, such as a brain aneurysm.

II. **Contraindications and Cautions**
   A. Contraindicated if the fetus has a bleeding disorder, such as hemophilia, thrombocytopenia, or osteogenesis imperfecta
   B. Vacuum is contraindicated at less than 34 weeks gestation
   C. Combined vacuum and forceps delivery is contraindicated.
   D. Midforceps are infrequently used.
   E. Shoulder dystocia is common in patients with diabetes or suspected macrosomia.

III. **Requirements Before Operative Vaginal Delivery**
   A. Pelvis must be adequate.
   B. Anesthesia or analgesia must be adequate.
   C. Urine must be emptied with catheter.
   D. Station must be more than +2 for low forceps and vacuum, and the cervix must be completely dilated and membranes ruptured.

IV. **Criteria for Types of Forceps Delivery**
   A. **Outlet Forceps**
      1. Scalp is visible at the introitus without separating labia.
      2. Fetal skull has reached pelvic floor.
      3. Sagittal suture is in the anteroposterior diameter or right or left occiput anterior or posterior position.
      4. Fetal head is at or on the perineum.
      5. Rotation is less than 45 degrees.
   B. **Low Forceps**
      1. Leading point of fetal skull is at +2 or more, and not on the pelvic floor.
      2. Rotation is 45 degrees or less.
      3. Rotation is more than 45 degrees.

V. **Vacuum Delivery**
   A. Same indications, contraindications, and classifications as for forceps
   B. Avoid manual torque to the vacuum cup.
   C. Limit the vacuum detachments (pop-offs) to 3 or less. Maximum vacuum application time should be limited to 30 min.

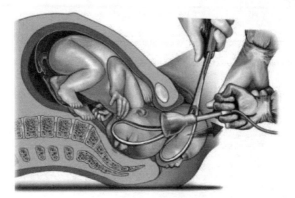

Figure: Vacuum and forceps delivery

Cesarean Delivery

Cesarean delivery is the most frequently performed surgery. The cesarean rate is 32% of all births.

I. **Common Indications for Cesarean** include previous cesarean, nonreassuring fetal heart rate patterns, labor dystocia, multiple gestation, macrosomia, preeclampsia, and breech presentation.

II. **Timing of Elective Cesarean Delivery**
   A. Elective cesarean delivery for prior low transverse uterine incision should be performed at 39–40 gestational weeks when the fetal lungs are mature. Amniocentesis to confirm maturity lung fetal is advised if elective cesarean delivery is to be performed before 39 weeks.
   B. Patients with a history of prior classical cesarean should receive a repeat cesarean delivery at 36–37 weeks.
   C. Patients with a prior complicated myomectomy should receive cesarean delivery at 37–38 weeks.
   D. Blood type and screen and hemoglobin and hematocrit before surgery

III. **Prophylactic Antibiotics for Cesarean**
   A. Cefazolin (Ancef) 1 gram IV, or 2 grams for women with BMI >30 or weight >100 kg within 60 min before skin incision.
   B. Penicillin hypersensitivity with prior anaphylaxis, angioedema, respiratory distress or urticaria is managed with gentamicin 1.5 mg/kg plus clindamycin 600 mg.

IV. **Thromboprophylaxis for Cesarean Section**
   A. Cesarean is a risk factor of venous thromboembolism 0.9%.
   B. A mechanical thromboprophylaxis compression device is applied preoperatively and continue until the patient ambulates.
   C. For patients at high risk for venous thromboembolism (e.g., severe obesity, previous venous thromboembolism or immobility), use low molecular weight heparins, e.g., enoxaparin 40 mg qd or unfractionated heparin 5,000 units q12h. Delay injections until 12h after spinal anesthesia.

V. **Low Transverse vs. Midline Vertical Skin Incision**
   A. The low transverse incision is a 12–15 cm and 2–5 cm above pubic

symphysis. The low transverse is the most common incision for cesarean delivery.
   B. The midline vertical skin incision provides faster abdominal entry in repeat cesareans, results in less bleeding and nerve injury, and is easily extensible.
VI. **Pfannenstiel vs. Joel-Cohen Abdominal Entry**
   A. The Pfannenstiel entry involves separation of the fascia layer from rectus muscle.
   B. The Joel-Cohen entry uses blunt finger dissection into the abdominal cavity after incision of the fascia layer. The Joel-Cohen entry provides fast entry and less blood loss compared to the Pfannenstiel entry.
VII. **Uterine Incision**
   A. The low transverse incision is indicated for preterm delivery.
   B. Vertical midline and low vertical or classical incisions are used for very premature fetuses in transverse back-down position, anterior placenta previa or accreta, and very premature fetuses.
VIII. **Uterine Closure and Future Risk of Uterine Rupture during VBAC**
   A. The two-layer uterine closure has a decreased risk of uterine rupture or dehiscence.
IX. **Subcutaneous Closure**
   A. Closure of subcutaneous tissue is advised if the depth is more than 2 cm.
X. **Postoperative Care and Complications**
   A. Post cesarean delivery patients are discharged on post-op day 2–4. Staples are usually removed on post-op day 3 for transverse skin incisions and post-op day 5 for vertical skin incisions.
   B. Post-op complications include hemorrhage, endometritis, wound infection, thromboembolism, and urinary tract or bowel injuries.

Shoulder Dystocia

Shoulder dystocia occurs in 1.5% of vaginal deliveries.

I. **Definition for Shoulder Dystocia**
   A. Impaction of the anterior shoulder against the pubic symphysis after delivery of the head and failure of gentle downward traction to cause delivery.
   B. Head-to-body delivery time is more than 60 seconds.
II. **Risk Factors for Shoulder dystocia**
   A. Prior shoulder dystocia, fetal macrosomia, diabetes, post-term, male fetus, advanced maternal age, excessive weight gain, abnormal pelvis, and multiparity
   B. Abnormal first-stage labor, arrest disorder, labor augmentation with oxytocin, and instrument delivery.
III. **Fetal Macrosomia**
   A. Macrosomia is a fetal weight ≥4,500 grams.
   B. Macrosomia is associated with shoulder dystocia, Erb's palsy, postpartum hemorrhage, and perineal laceration.
   C. Prenatal diagnosis of macrosomia is highly inaccurate. Ultrasound is inaccurate if >4,500 grams.
IV. **Prevention of Shoulder Dystocia**
   A. Perform cesarean if estimated fetal weight is >5,000 grams in women without diabetes and >4,500 grams in women with diabetes.
   B. Avoid vacuum or forceps if prior shoulder dystocia, macrosomia, or diabetes are present.
   C. Consider cesarean if the patient had a prior shoulder dystocia.

V. **Treatment of Shoulder Dystocia**
   A. **McRoberts maneuver**: Flex the thighs against the abdomen.
   B. **Call for help.**
   C. **Suprapubic pressure.**
   D. **Delivery of the posterior arm** is the most effective maneuver for shoulder dystocia.
      1. **Woods maneuver** is the insertion a hand into the posterior vagina and rotation of the posterior shoulder in a clockwise or counterclockwise direction.
      2. **Rubin maneuver** pushes the posterior or anterior shoulder in the direction of the fetal chest to adduct the shoulders.
      3. **Deliberate clavicular fracture**
      4. **Zavanelli maneuver** (push back the delivered fetal head into the birth canal and perform cesarean section), or symphysiotomy may also be attempted.

VI. **Complications Associated with Shoulder Dystocia**
   A. **Fetal Brachial Plexus Palsy**
      1. Brachial plexus palsy is caused by excessive downward fetal traction.
      2. Upper arm palsy (Erb-Duchenne) is the most frequent brachial palsy. Upper arm palsy is caused by injury to C5–C7
      3. Lower arm palsy (Klumpke) results from injury to C8–T1 and is associated with Horner's syndrome.
      4. Most brachial plexus palsies resolve before discharge. 90% resolve by 1 year
   B. **Fetal Fractures**
      1. Clavicular fractures most commonly occur after a normal vaginal delivery.
      2. Humeral fractures are infrequent and can occur during delivery of the posterior arm.

Vaginal Birth after Cesarean

I. **Risks and Benefits of Vaginal Birth after Cesarean**
   A. All the births have a risk of maternal hemorrhage and transfusion, infection, thromboembolism, hysterectomy, and fetal and maternal death.
   B. Trial of labor after previous cesarean delivery is associated with fewer complications. But a failed trial of labor after Cesarean is associated with more complications. Complete uterine rupture may result in hemorrhage, cord prolapse, and extrusion of the fetus and placenta into the abdominal cavity. Incomplete rupture or uterine dehiscence occurs when the uterine muscle is separated but visceral serosa remains intact.
   C. The success rate of is 80%.

II. **Risks for Uterine Rupture with Trial of Labor after Cesarean**
   A. The risk of uterine rupture is 0.5% for low transverse uterine incisions
   B. The risk of uterine rupture is 4% for classical and T-shaped incisions

III. **Candidates for Trial of Labor After Cesarean**
   A. One previous low-transverse cesarean delivery
   B. Prior low vertical incision

IV. **Contraindications for Trial of Labor After Cesarean**
   A. Prior classical or T-shaped incision or extensive uterine surgery
   B. Previous uterine rupture
   C. Medical or obstetric disorder

V. **Factors Favoring Vaginal Birth After Cesarean**
   A. Prior vaginal delivery
   B. Previous successful VBAC

C. Favorable cervix
D. Spontaneous onset of labor
E. Breech presentation was the indication for the previous cesarean
F. Maternal age <35–40
G. Interdelivery interval >18 months
H. Fetal birth weight <4,000 grams
I. Maternal weight <300 lbs

VI. **Labor Management for TOLAC**
A. Epidural anesthesia can be used for pain management.
B. Severe variable decelerations or late decelerations are the most sensitive indicators for uterine rupture.
C. Labor induction is associated with a higher rate of uterine rupture and lower rate of success.
D. Cervical ripening with prostaglandins increases the risk of uterine rupture. Labor induction with oxytocin raises the risk of uterine rupture.
E. Mechanical cervical ripening with a Foley catheter can be used for labor induction.
F. Labor Augmentation with low dose of oxytocin (≤20 mU/min) for labor augmentation does not increase the risk of uterine rupture.

External Cephalic Version

I. **Clinical Evaluation**
A. Breech presentation occurs in 3% of term deliveries. Planned singleton breech delivery is contraindicated because of elevated risk of neonatal complications (5%).
B. Ultrasound is used to confirm fetal lie or presentation if breech is suspected. Abdominal palpation with Leopold's maneuver is not sensitive (sensitivity 57%). Vaginal exam is useful in detection of cephalic presentation.
C. External cephalic version is external manipulation through the abdominal wall to turn the fetus from breech to cephalic position.
D. **Timing and Success Rate**
1. External cephalic version is performed at 36 to 38 weeks of gestation if the fetus is in the breech presentation.
2. Success rate is 60%.

II. **Contraindications to External Cephalic Version**
A. Placenta previa
B. Placental abruption
C. Non-reassuring fetal heart rate
D. Fetal or uterine anomaly
E. Hyperextension of the fetal head

III. **Procedure**
A. Obtain informed consent. Ensure that an emergency cesarean could be performed if needed. Confirm gestational age ≥36 completed weeks. Perform ultrasound to ensure that there are no contraindications, such as placenta previa. Confirm that the fetal heart tracing is reassuring. Empty the bladder and give terbutaline 0.25 mg SC or IV for uterine relaxation.
B. Apply ultrasound gel to keep the abdomen slick. First use forward roll. Use back flip if forward roll fails. Stop the procedure if fetal bradycardia or excessive discomfort develops.
C. After external cephalic version, monitor fetal heart rates to ensure that FHT is reassuring. Give RhoGAM if Rh negative and patient did not receive RhoGAM at 28 weeks.

IV. **Complications of External Cephalic Version**
A. Fetal heart rate decelerations, preterm labor, placental abruption, uterine

rupture, and fetal demise.
B. Fetal-maternal hemorrhage may occur in 2.4%.

Assessment of the Newborn

I. APGAR Scores
A. Low Apgar scores at 1 minute require neonatal resuscitation but do not
predict long-term neurological outcome.
B. Apgar scores of less than 3 at 5 minutes or later are associated with neurological dysfunction or cerebral palsy.
C. Apgar scores of <7 at 5 minutes are associated with cognitive impairment.

APGAR Score Assessment of the Neonate			
	0	1	2
Appearance	Blue all over	Extremities blue, trunk pink	Pink all over
Pulse	-	<100	>100
Grimace (reaction to suctioning)	No reaction	Facial grimace	Sneeze or cry
Activity	No move-ment	Only slight flexing of ex-tremities	Moving normally
Respiratory effort	None	Slow breathing, weak cry	Good breathing, strong cry

II. Umbilical Cord Blood pH and Gases
A. Umbilical cord blood pH and gases provide an objective evaluation of
fetal hypoxia and acidemia.
B. A blood sample should be obtained from the arteries. The arterial values
reflect fetal acid-base status more accurately than venous values. Venous values reflect the placental acid-base status.

III. Collection Techniques
A. The cord should be doubly clamped after delivery because neonatal
breathing can alter cord acid-base values.
B. Collect a sample from the artery first.
C. Consider cord blood analysis for meconium staining, abnormal fetal heart
rate patterns, low Apgar scores, preterm birth, breech delivery, severe intrauterine growth restriction and chorioamnionitis.

IV. Cerebral Palsy
A. Cerebral palsy is an upper motor neuron brain injury characterized by
hyperactive tendon reflexes, increased muscle tone, and spasticity.
B. Cerebral palsy is associated with low intelligence and seizure disorders.

Postpartum Care

Postpartum Hemorrhage

Postpartum hemorrhage is the leading cause of maternal death and affects 1% of deliveries. Postpartum hemorrhage is defined as ≥500 ml of blood loss with a vaginal delivery or ≥1,000 ml with cesarean delivery.

I. Etiology
A. Uterine atony is the most frequent cause of PPH. Risk factors for PPH include grand multiparity, multiple gestation, prolonged labor, prolonged oxytocin, chorioamnionitis, and tocolytics.

B. Other etiologies of postpartum hemorrhage include vaginal or cervical laceration, retained placenta, placenta accreta, uterine inversion, and bleeding disorders.

C. Placenta accreta is the most frequent cause of persistent postpartum hemorrhage and is the most common indication for peri-partum hysterectomy.

D. Retained placenta may result in delayed PPH.

II. Prevention of Post Partum Hemorrhage
A. Administration of 40 units of oxytocin after delivery of the placenta prevents PPH.

III. Management of Postpartum Hemorrhage
A. The placenta, membranes, or blood clots should be removed from uterus, and then the uterus should be massaged bimanually. The bladder should be emptied with catheter.

B. Monitor blood loss, vital signs, and urine output.

C. Place two 16 to 18-gauge IV lines. Infuse 2 L of warm normal saline at a 3:1 ratio to the estimated blood loss.

D. The patient should be moved to the operating room if bleeding continues after uterotonic agents are given.

E. Oxytocin (Pitocin)
  1. 10–40 units in 1,000 ml LR or NS IV infusion; 10 units may be given IM or by direct injection into uterus through the abdomen or cervix if an IV is not present.
  2. Side effects of oxytocin include water intoxication and hyponatremia. Oxytocin may cause hypotension if given by IV bolus.

F. Methylergonovine (Methergine)
  1. 0.2 mg IM
  2. Side effects: hypertension, nausea, vomiting, and chest pain. Contraindicated in hypertension or vascular diseases

G. 15-Methyl PG F_{2a} (carboprost, Hemabate)
  1. 0.25 mg IM or intramyometrial injection every 15 minutes; maximum 8 doses.
  2. Side effects of 15-methyl PG F_{2a} include nausea, vomiting, diarrhea, fever, bronchospasm and hypertension. 15-methyl PG F_{2a} is contraindicated in asthma, heart, lung, renal or liver disease

H. Transfusion
1. If the estimated blood loss is more than 1,500 ml, heart rate ≥110, blood pressure ≤85/45 mmHg or O_2sat <95%, PRBCs should be transfused. Hemoglobin and hematocrit do not reflect acute blood loss.
2. If postpartum hemorrhage does not respond to oxytocin and one additional uterotonic agent, blood loss is >1,000 ml, 2 units of PRBC should be infused.
3. **Packed Red Blood Cells**
   a) Indications for PRBCs include acute blood loss, symptomatic anemia, and hemoglobin <7 g/dl
   b) 300–350 ml/unit.
   c) One unit of pRBCs will increase the hemoglobin by 1 g/dl or hematocrit by 3–4%
4. **Fresh Frozen Plasma**
   a) Fresh frozen plasma contains all coagulation factors
   b) Fresh frozen plasma is indicated if more than 2 units of PRBCs were given, or if INR >1.5 seconds
   c) 250 ml/unit. Must be ABO compatible
5. **Platelets**
   a) Platelets are indicated if the platelet count is <50,000/ mm^3
   b) Contains 400 ml plasma
   c) One unit raises platelets by 4,500/mm^3.
6. **Massive Transfusion Protocol**
   a) Massive transfusion protocol should be initiated in the following situations:
      (1) Total blood loss of more than 1,500 ml and bleeding continues
      (2) Continued bleeding after transfusion 2 units of PRBC
      (3) Unstable vital signs
      (4) Disseminated intravascular coagulation
   b) The massive transfusion protocol is 6 units of PRBC, 6 units of fresh frozen plasma, and 6-units of platelets. Transfuse plasma to RBCs in a 1:1 ratio.
   c) CBC, INR, aPTT, fibrinogen, chem 12, ABG should be checked every 60 minutes
7. **Adverse Reactions to Blood Transfusion**
   a) Acute reactions to blood transfusion include fever (1.5%) and urticaria (3%). Hemolysis, anaphylaxis, and acute lung injury are infrequent.
   b) Massive transfusion may cause metabolic acidosis, hypocalcemia, and hyperkalemia. Hypocalcemia should be corrected with 10% calcium gluconate 10 ml IV or 10% calcium chloride 5 ml IV per 500 ml of blood.

I. Surgical Treatment of Postpartum Hemorrhage
1. **Uterine Curettage**
   a) If retained tissue is the source of bleeding, uterine curettage will stop the bleeding. A large curette is used to gently remove the product of conception. Excessively vigorous curettage may cause uterine scarring and infertility.
2. **Uterine Packing or Tamponade**
   a) Uterine packing using gauze is not frequently used due to the risk of concealed bleeding and endometritis.
   b) The Bakri Tamponade Balloon controls hemorrhage from lower uterine segment. The balloon is filled with normal saline. The balloon is removed within 24 hours.

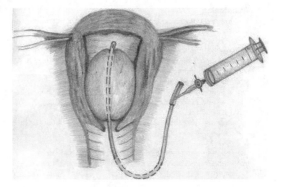

Figure: The Bakri tamponade balloon

3. **Selective Arterial Embolization**
   a) Selective arterial embolization is minimally invasive.
   b) The patient needs to be stabilized being sent to the radiology suite.
4. **Arterial Ligation**
   a) Bilateral uterine artery ligation and bilateral utero-ovarian artery ligation can be performed.
   b) Ligation of internal iliac arteries is technically difficult.
5. **Uterine Compression Suture**
   a) The B-Lynch suture for uterine compression was a success rate of 75%.
   b) Complications include uterine necrosis, pyometra, and myometrial defects.
6. **Hysterectomy**
   a) Hysterectomy is indicated when other measures do not control bleeding.
   b) Supracervical is easy to perform rapidly and causes less injury to bladder and ureter.
7. **Uterine Inversion**
   a) Complete or incomplete uterine inversion may cause massive bleeding and shock.
   b) Treatment of uterine inversion is manual replacement of the uterine fundus with the placenta attached. Tocolytics include terbutaline 0.25 mg IV, magnesium sulfate 4g IV, or nitroglycerin 0.4–0.8 mg sublingual or 50–200 µg IV.
8. **Postpartum Anemia**
   a) Symptoms of anemia include headache, light-headedness, tachycardia, and syncope.
   b) Give $FeSO_4$ 325 mg tid with vitamin C 500 mg tid to promote absorption of iron.
   c) Transfusion for postpartum anemia is infrequently needed when the hemoglobin is more than 10 g/dL. Transfusion is always indicated when hemoglobin is <6 g/dL. When the hemoglobin is 6–10 g/dl, transfusion should be based on symptoms, pulse, blood pressure, and skin temperature.

Postpartum Fever

I. **Causes of Postpartum Fever**
   A. Womb: Endomyometritis is the most common cause of puerperal fever.
   B. Wind: pneumonia or atelectasis
   C. Water: urinary tract infection
   D. Wound: wound infection
   E. Walk: deep vein thrombosis, pulmonary embolism, or venous thrombo-phlebitis
   F. Weaning: breast engorgement or mastitis
   G. Wonder drugs: drug fever

Endometritis

I. **Diagnosis**
   A. **Fever:** temperature ≥38.0° C after delivery
   B. **Foul-smelling lochia**, abdominal and fundal tenderness and elevated WBC

II. **Treatment of Endometritis**
   A. Continue antibiotics for 24 hours after afebrile. Oral antibiotics are not needed after discharge.
   B. **Antibiotic Regimens of Endometritis**
      1. Clindamycin 900 mg q8h and gentamicin 5 mg/kg IV once a day.
      2. For enterococci infection, add ampicillin 2g q6h.
      3. **Other Antibiotic Regimens**
         a) Ampicillin/sulbactam (Unasyn) 3g IV q6h
         b) Ticarcillin-clavulanate (Timentin) 3.1g IV q4–6h
         c) Piperacillin-tazobactam (Zosyn) 3.375–4.5 g IV q6h
   C. **Oral regimen:** Augmentin (Amoxicillin-clavulanate) 875 mg q12h

Puerperal Septic Pelvic Thrombophlebitis

Puerperal septic pelvic thrombophlebitis is an infection of the ovarian venous plexus.

I. **Diagnosis**
   A. Persistent fever >5 days despite adequate antibiotic coverage.
   B. Pelvic CT or MRI is diagnostic for ovarian venous thrombosis.

II. **Treatment**
   A. Continue antibiotics for 2 days after afebrile.
   B. Systemic anticoagulation is frequently used.
   C. Stop anticoagulation when antibiotics are discontinued.

Amniotic Fluid Embolism

I. **Clinical Evaluation**
   A. Amniotic fluid embolism causes 7.5% of maternal deaths.
   B. Induction of labor and cesarean deliveries are risk factors for AFE.
   C. Amniotic fluid embolism presents with maternal hemorrhage (65%), hypotension (63%), dyspnea (62%), coagulopathy (62%), premonitory restlessness, agitation, numbness, tingling (47%), and acute fetal compromise (43%).

II. **Treatment**
   A. Treatment of amniotic fluid embolism is oxygen, cardiopulmonary support, and transfusion of blood components to correct coagulopathy.
   B. Perimortem cesarean delivery may be needed.

Postpartum Care

I. **General Postpartum Care**
   A. Ambulate. Use stool softeners.
   B. Resume intercourse 2–4 weeks postpartum.
II. **Cesarean Wound Care**
   A. If the incision is transverse, remove staples on post-op day 3 and apply Steri-strips.
   B. If the incision is vertical, remove staples after 5 days, and apply strips-strips.
III. **Hemorrhoid Care**
   A. Increase fiber intake and use a stool softener.
   B. Topical OTC agents include 1% or 2.5% hydrocortisone cream for itching; 1% pramoxine ointment, gel, foam, or cream for pain.
IV. **Breastfeeding**
   A. Initiate breastfeeding within the first hour after delivery and 8–12 times a day on demand. Milk production becomes copious 1–5 day postpartum.
   B. **Contraindications to Breastfeeding**
      1. Positive HIV
      2. Untreated active TB, active varicella or active herpes breast lesions
      3. Currently being treated for breast cancer
      4. Maternal drug abuse
      5. Infant with galactosemia
      6. Chemotherapy using cytotoxic drugs, such as methotrexate, cyclophosphamide, cyclosporine, doxorubicin, and radioactive compounds
   C. **Medications During Lactation**
   D. Antianxiety drugs, antidepressants, and neuroleptic drugs may be of concern." Other drugs in this category include amiodarone, lamotrigine, metoclopramide, metronidazole, and tinidazole.
   E. **Common Problems Associated with Breastfeeding**
      1. **Engorgement**
         a) Engorgement occurs 72 hours postpartum and at weaning.
         b) Emptying the breasts frequently prevents and treats engorgement.
         c) Acetaminophen, ibuprofen, and cool compresses, or ice packs relieve breast pain.
      2. **Mastitis**
         a) Mastitis is caused by Staphylococcus aureus, streptococcus, or E. coli.
         b) Mastitis causes a hard, red, tender, and swollen area with fever, chills, myalgia, and malaise.
         c) Dicloxacillin or cephalexin 500 mg po q6h for 10–14 days. If no response within 24–48h, switch to amoxicillin/clavulanate (Augmentin).
         d) MRSA is treated with trimethoprim-sulfamethoxazole DS 1 to 2 tabs PO 2 times a day or clindamycin 300 mg PO q6h. For severe MRSA infection, treat with vancomycin 1 g IV q12h.
      3. **Breast Abscess**
         a) Fluctuant breast abscesses are drained by needle aspiration. Ultrasound may be used to guide aspiration.
         b) Perform incision and drainage if aspiration is not effective.
         c) Breastfeeding should be continued.

V. Contraception
A. Contraception for Non-breastfeeding Women
1. Ovulation can occur 3–4 weeks after delivery.
2. Progestin-only pills, injections and contraceptive implants can be started postpartum.
3. Combined OCs may be started 3–4 weeks postpartum after hyper-coagulability resolves.

B. Contraception for Breastfeeding Women
1. **Non-hormonal Methods.** Condoms, copper intrauterine system, and postpartum bilateral tubal ligation.
2. **Hormonal Methods**
   a) Progestin-only pills are started 2–3 weeks postpartum. Pills include Micronor, Nor-once a day, Nora BE, Errin, and Ovrette.
   b) Depo medroxyprogesterone, progesterone intrauterine system, or an etonogestrel implant may be initiated 6 weeks postpartum.

VI. Depression
A. Depressive disorder occurs in 10% of pregnant women, and half of these may have major depression.
B. DSM-5 Diagnostic Criteria for Major Depression
1. ≥ 5 following symptoms present for ≥ 2 consecutive weeks. At least 1 symptom is 1) depressed mood or 2) loss of interest or pleasure.
2. Depressed mood most of the day, nearly every day
3. Markedly diminished interest or pleasure
4. Significant weight loss or weight gain
5. Insomnia/hypersomnia
6. Psychomotor retardation or agitation
7. Fatigue or loss of energy
8. Feeling of worthlessness or inappropriate guilt
9. Diminished ability to think or concentrate, or indecisiveness
10. Recurrent thoughts of death or suicide

C. Diagnostic Criteria for Dysthymic disorder
1. Depressed mood for ≥ 2 years. Accompanied by ≥ 2 of the following symptoms.
2. Decreased or increased appetite
3. Insomnia or hypersomnia
4. Fatigue or low energy
5. Low self esteem
6. Poor concentration or difficulty making decisions
7. Feeling" s of hopelessness

D. Diagnostic Criteria for Minor Depression
1. 2 to 4 symptoms of major depression have been present for ≥ 2 weeks. At least 1 symptom is depressed mood or loss of interest or pleasure.

VII. Treatment of Depression in Pregnancy
A. Patients with a major depressive disorder, psychosis, bipolar, or a serious suicide attempt should continue to take antidepressant medications during pregnancy.
B. Selective serotonin-reuptake inhibitors are safer and better tolerated than TCAs and MAO inhibitors.
C. Bupropion (Wellbutrin). Category C; XL 150 mg qAM; SR 100 mg 2 times a day. Not first-line drug. Useful for smoking cessation
D. Sertraline (Zoloft) 50 mg qd
E. Fluoxetine (Prozac). Associated with ventricular septal defect; 20 mg qAM
F. Escitalopram (Lexapro) 10 mg qd
G. Venlafaxine (Effexor). Category C; 37.5 mg 2 times a day
H. Paroxetine (Paxil). Possible cardiac malformations; 20 mg qAM

I. **Effect of Antidepressants on Birth Outcomes**
    1. Newborn adaptation symptoms may include tachypnea, hypoglyce-
        mia, irritability, temperature instability or seizure. Symptoms resolve
        within 2 weeks after delivery.
    2. Persistent pulmonary hypertension of the newborn has a six-fold rela-
        tive risk (0.1%) in neonates exposed to selective serotonin-reuptake
        inhibitors.
    3. First-trimester use of paroxetine may be associated with cardiac mal-
        formation.

VIII. **Postpartum Blues and Postpartum Depression**
    A. Postpartum blues are manifested by mild mood swings with sadness,
        crying, insomnia, anxiety, and poor concentration. Postpartum blues
        has an onset and resolution within 2 weeks of delivery. Treatment is re-
        assurance.
    B. Postpartum depression is severe major depressive disorder within 4
        weeks postpartum. Postpartum depression has a prevalence 5%.

Prenatal Care

Maternal Physiology

I. Cardiopulmonary Changes of Pregnancy
  A. Nasal stuffiness and epistaxis occur in pregnancy because of mucosal edema
  B. The ventilation rate and tidal volume increase, resulting in a mild respiratory alkalosis. The reduced maternal PCO_2 from hyperventilation facilitates CO_2 transfer from the fetus to the mother.
  C. A systolic murmur along the left sternal border can be heard in 90% of women during pregnancy. A third heart sound is often audible. Systolic murmur that is louder than a grade 2/4 is abnormal. Diastolic murmurs are also abnormal.

II. Genitourinary System
  A. Normal pregnancy causes urinary frequency, nocturia, and stress incontinence. Urinary stasis and asymptomatic bacteriuria occurs in 8% of pregnancies
  B. Renal plasma flow rises by 30% by 20 weeks.
  C. Decreased creatinine (abnormal if >0.8)

III. Hematologic System
  A. Plasma volume rises by 50% during pregnancy, resulting in hemodilution. The WBC increases 5,600 to 12,200/mm^3 in second and third trimesters.
  B. The normal hemoglobin of 12–16 g/dl, drops to 10.5 g/dl in second trimester. Pregnancy reduces iron and ferritin. Pregnancy causes elevated transferrin.

IV. Coagulation Factors. VII, VIII, X, fibrinogen, von Willebrand factor, plasminogen activator inhibitor-1 and plasminogen activator inhibitor-2 increase during pregnancy

V. Endocrine
  A. hCG is detectable at 7 days before the expected menses. hCG doubles every 31 hours to a peak hCG of 100,000 at 10 weeks. The hCG declines to 10,000 at term.
  B. Progesterone from the ovaries maintains the early pregnancy. Progesterone should be administered if ovarian progesterone production is compromised before 9–10 weeks.
  C. Thyroid size, total thyroxine, and thyroxine-binding globulin increase in pregnancy. The free thyroxine level remains normal in pregnancy.
  D. Elevated cortisol, aldosterone, insulin, and increased insulin receptors occur in pregnancy. Increased insulin resistance results from elevated hPL and prolactin

VI. Gastrointestinal System
  A. Pregnancy causes gastroesophageal reflex, constipation, hemorrhoids, and cholestasis

Routine Prenatal Care

I. Terminology of Pregnancy
  A. **Gravidity**
    1. Gravity is the number of times a woman has been pregnant
    2. Gravida is a woman who is or has been pregnant
    3. Primigravida is a woman in her first pregnancy
    4. Multigravida is a woman with >1 pregnancies

     5. Nulligravida is a woman who has never been pregnant

  B. **Parity**

    1. Parity is the number of times a women has given birth after 20-week gestation or given birth to an infant ≥500 grams

    2. Primipara is a woman who has delivered once at ≥20 weeks

    3. Multipara is a women who has delivered twice or more at ≥20 weeks

    4. Nullipara is a women who has never completed a pregnancy ≥20 weeks

II. Trimester

  A. First Trimester: 0–14 weeks

  B. Second Trimester: 14–28 weeks

  C. Third Trimester: 28 weeks to birth

III. G_nP_{TPAL}

  A. Gn is the total number of pregnancies

  B. T is the total number of term deliveries (≥37 weeks)

  C. P is the total number of preterm deliveries (20–37 weeks)

  D. A is the total number of abortions or miscarriages (<20 weeks)

  E. L is the total number of living children

IV. Estimation of Gestational Age

  A. Naegele's Rule: Estimated date of delivery (EDD) is calculated by adding 7 to the date of the first day of LMP and counting back 3 months.

  B. The ultrasound date should be used if the LMP is unreliable.

V. Fetal Development

  A. Fetal heart sounds are first heard at 11–12 weeks with a handheld Doppler.

  B. Ultrasound, the gestational sac is visible at 5–6 weeks. The fetal pole and cardiac activity are visible at 7–8 weeks.

  C. Fetal movement is usually first felt by the patient at 17–18 weeks (quickening).

  D. The fundus is palpable at the pubic symphysis at 12 weeks. The fundus is midway between symphysis and umbilicus at 16 weeks. The fundus is at the umbilicus at 20 weeks.

VI. Prenatal Care Visits

  A. Patients should have clinic appointments every 4 weeks before 28 weeks; every 2 weeks between 28–36 weeks. Then weekly after.

  B. Check the blood pressure, weight, fundal height, fetal heart tones, and urine dipstick at every prenatal clinic appointment.

  C. Fetal movement counting is not routinely recommended.

  D. A cervix exam should be performed if the patient has contractions, bleeding, discharge, or leakage of fluid.

  E. **First Prenatal Visit**

    1. History and physical, including pelvic and breast exam

    2. Initial labs: blood type and Rh type, antibody screen, hemoglobin and hematocrit, cervical cytology, rubella, varicella, VDRL/RPR, urine culture, HBsAg, and HIV.

    3. Optional labs: PPD or QuantiFERON for TB screening, gonorrhea and Chlamydia tests, and screening for genetic diseases (cystic fibrosis, α and β thalassemia, sickle cell disease, or Tay-Sachs disease).

  F. **8–20 Weeks**

    1. Ultrasound is done at 18–20 weeks for fetal anatomy survey.

    2. Quadruple testing (AFP, total hCG, uE3, and inhibin A) is done at 15 to 20 weeks

  G. **24–28 Weeks**

    1. Screen for gestational diabetes with hemoglobin-A1c.

    2. Give RhIG if Rh negative at 28 weeks.

    3. Hemoglobin and hematocrit

H. **32–36 Weeks**
   1. The fetal presentation does not need to be assessed before 36 weeks because the fetal presentation will often change before delivery.
   2. Obtain a group B streptococcus culture at 35 to 37 weeks.
   3. Hemoglobin and hematocrit
   4. Ultrasound, HIV test, VDRL/RPR, and gonococcus/Chlamydia

VII. **Common Concerns During Pregnancy**
   A. **Weight Gain in Pregnancy**
      1. Women with a BMI <18.5 (underweight) should gain 12.5–18 kg or 28–40 lb
      2. Women with a BMI 18.5–24.9 (normal weight) should gain 11.5–16 kg or 25–35 lb
      3. Women with a BMI 25–29.9 (overweight) should gain 7–11.5 kg or 15–25 lb
      4. Women with a BMI ≥30 (obese) should gain 5–9 kg or 11–20 lb
   B. **Diet and Vitamins**. A prenatal vitamin should be taken once a day. Prenatal vitamins contain 27 mg of iron, 0.4 mg of folic acid, and 5,000 IU of vitamin A.
   C. **Alcohol** is teratogen and no safe threshold has been established. Alcohol should be discontinued before pregnancy. Fetal alcohol syndrome consists of craniofacial, cardiac, spinal and brain defects, and behavior disturbances.
   D. **Tobacco** is associated with preterm labor, low birth weight, fetal growth restriction, placental abruption, cleft lip and palate, and vascular disturbances
   E. **Pregnancy-associated Symptoms**. Common symptoms during pregnancy include nausea and vomiting, heartburn, hemorrhoids, constipation, urinary frequency and incontinence, back pain, sciatica, round ligament pain, carpal tunnel syndrome, restless leg syndrome, and syncope
   F. **Nausea and Vomiting in Pregnancy**
      1. Nausea and vomiting usually start at 4 weeks and resolves before 16 weeks. About 85% of pregnant women have nausea and vomiting.
      2. Hyperemesis gravidarum is present in 2% of pregnancies with persistent vomiting, ketonuria, and ≥5% of weight loss.
      3. **Treatment of Nausea and Vomiting in Pregnancy**
         a) Step 1: Vitamin B6 (pyridoxine) 25 mg PO q6–8h
         b) Step 2: Vitamin B6 and doxylamine 12.5 mg (half tab of Unisom) PO q6–8h
         c) Step 3: Vitamin B6 and doxylamine q6–8h and promethazine (Phenergan) 12.5–25 mg q4h PO or PR, or dimenhydrinate (Dramamine) 50–100 mg q4–6h PO or PR
         d) Step 4:
            (1) Add metoclopramide (Reglan) 5–10 mg every 8 hours IM or PO, or promethazine 12.5–25 mg IM, or trimethobenzamide (Tigan) 200 mg every 6–8 hours per rectum
            (2) If dehydrated, give IV fluid. For prolonged vomiting, consider IV thiamine 100 mg, folic acid 1 mg, multivitamins 1 ample, and $MgSO_4$ 2 g in 1 L of lactated ringers. Add promethazine 12.5–25 mg IV q4h, or dimenhydrinate IV q4–6h, or metoclopramide 5–10 mg IV.
         e) Step 5: Add methylprednisolone 16 mg q8h PO or IV or ondansetron (Zofran) 8 mg IV q12h. Ondansetron is a serotonin 5–HT3 receptor antagonist; 4–8 mg PO once a day or 3 times a day.

VIII. Routine Laboratory Testing

    A. First prenatal visit lab tests include hematocrit and hemoglobin levels, urinalysis and culture, blood type and antibody screen, rubella immunity, syphilis, HBsAg, HIV, cervical cytology, and chlamydia.

    B. Tuberculosis screening with PPD or QuantiFERON is indicated in high-risk populations.

    C. Cystic fibrosis screening should be offered to Caucasians and persons with a family history of cystic fibrosis.

    D. Repeat hemoglobin and hematocrit and screen for chlamydia, syphilis, and HIV in the third trimester.

    E. Group B streptococcus screening should be performed at 35 to 37 weeks.

IX. Immunization in Pregnancy

    A. **Live Attenuated Virus Vaccine**

        1. Measles, mumps, rubella (MMR) and varicella are contraindicated during pregnancy due to a theoretical risk to the fetus.

        2. If a pregnant women is non-immune to MMR, a single dose MMR vaccine is given at 4 weeks postpartum.

    B. **Inactivated Influenza Virus Vaccine**. Give one dose to all patients during the flu season regardless of trimester of pregnancy.

    C. **Tetanus, Diphtheria and Pertussis Vaccine**

        1. Give Td booster after 20 weeks of gestation if the patient has not received a Td vaccination within the last 10 years or TDaP if she has not been previously vaccinated with TDaP.

        2. If a pregnant woman has never been vaccinated against tetanus, she should receive three vaccinations at 0, 4 weeks, and 6–12 months. One dose of Tdap should be given after 20 weeks of gestation. If not given during pregnancy, Tdap should be administered immediately postpartum.

    D. **Hepatitis A and B Vaccines**

        1. Hepatitis A and B vaccines should be administered to women at risk of infections. Immunoglobulins may also be used for postexposure prophylaxis.

        2. Three doses of hepatitis B vaccines are given at 0, 1, and 6 months.

        3. Two doses of hepatitis A vaccines are given 6 months apart.

Prenatal Diagnosis

I. Fetal Aneuploidy

    A. Fetal aneuploidy is associated with a 4 –fold increase from age 35 to 40; there is a 10–fold increase in the incidence of aneuploidy from age 40 to 48 years.

    B. **Noninvasive Screening Tests with Maternal Serum Analytes**

        1. Many positive screening tests are false positive. Error in gestational dating is a common reason for a positive serum analyte test.

        2. Further testing with fetal karyotype is indicated if screening test is positive.

    C. **Second Trimester (15–17 weeks)**: Quadruple screening (AFP, total hCG, uE3, and inhibin A) has an aneuploidy detection rate of 81%

    D. **Maternal Plasma-based Fetal DNA Testing**

        1. Highly sensitive and specific. Specificity 100%. Sensitivity 100% for trisomy 21, 97.2% for trisomy 18, and 78.6% for trisomy 13

        2. Maternal plasma-based fetal DNA testing may replace serum analytes for aneuploidy in the future.

II. Invasive Diagnostic Tests

    A. Invasive diagnostic tests are available to women of all ages.

   B. Patients with increased risk of fetal aneuploidy includes those with previous fetus or child with autosomal trisomy or sex chromosome abnormality, structural anomalies on ultrasound, parental carrier of chromosome translocation or inversion, parental aneuploidy or mosaicism for aneuploidy.

   C. **Amniocentesis** is performed at 15–20 weeks with fetal loss <1 in 300-500.

   D. **Chorionic Villus Sampling**

      1. CVS is performed after 9 completed weeks

      2. The fetal loss rate with CVS is the same as for amniocentesis.

      3. Fetal limb reduction and oromandibular defects are rare

III. Neural Tube Defects

   A. Neural tube defect screening with maternal serum AFP is measured at 15–20 weeks.

   B. Sensitivity 80–90%. Positive predictive value is 2–6%. The screen positive rate is 3%

   C. Fetal ultrasound and amniocentesis should be performed if the MSAFP is abnormal.

   D. **Other Conditions Associated with Elevated AFP** include multiple gestation, incorrect due date (AFP rises with gestational age), fetal demise, fetal-maternal hemorrhage, placental abnormalities, uterine anomalies, maternal dermoid cyst and hepatoma, omphalocele, gastroschisis, congenital nephrosis, sacrococcygeal teratoma, and triploidy

Drugs and Radiation in Pregnancy

I. **Drugs Suspected or Proven to be Human Teratogens:** ACE inhibitors, alcohol, androgens, busulfan, carbamazepine, coumarins, cyclophosphamide, danazol, etretinate, isotretinoin, lithium, methimazole, misoprostol, methotrexate, penicillamine, phenytoin, radioactive iodine, and valproic acid

II. **Antiepileptics and Antidepressants**

   A. Valproic acid during pregnancy may cause **spina bifida**, atrial septal defect, cleft palate, hypospadias, polydactyly, and craniosynostosis.

   B. Lamotrigine (Lamictal) and levetiracetam (Keppra) are safe in pregnancy.

III. **Sedatives**. Most benzodiazepines and barbitals are contraindicated in pregnancy Buspirone, zolpidem (Ambien), and propofol are safe in pregnancy.

IV. **Psychiatric Medications**

   A. Second-generation antipsychotics are safe in pregnancy. Antipsychotics are associated with neonatal extrapyramidal symptoms or withdrawal symptoms. Clozapine is safe and the other antipsychotics are category C.

   B. Lithium is associated with cardiovascular defects in the first trimester. Lamotrigine is often used for maintenance therapy for bipolar disorder.

V. **Cardiovasculars and Antihypertensives**

   A. ACE inhibitors and angiotensin II receptor antagonists may cause fetal renal tubular dysplasia, intrauterine growth restriction, oligohydramnios, and pulmonary hypoplasia.

   B. Neonatal thrombocytopenia is associated with thiazides but not with furosemide. Avoid diuretics in pregnancy.

   C. HMG-CoA reductase inhibitors (Statins) are associated with CNS and limb defects.

   D. All calcium channel blockers are category C. Amiodarone may cause fetal hyper- or hypothyroidism.

VI. Analgesics
 A. Aspirin in low-dosage is safe. Large aspirin doses is associated with an elevated risk of fetal bleeding, intrauterine growth restriction, premature closure of the ductus, gastroschisis, and intestinal atresia.
 B. NSAIDs may cause spontaneous abortion and may cause constriction of ductus arteriosus and neonatal pulmonary hypertension.
 C. Acetaminophen is safe, but hepatotoxic in overdose.
 D. Narcotics are associated with neonatal withdrawal syndrome.
VII. Antineoplastics. Asparaginase, dacarbazine, dactinomycin, and interferon are category C.
VIII. Antibiotics. Quinolones may cause bone and cartilage damage. Doxycycline may cause dental staining. Otonephrotoxicity has been reported with streptomycin.

Ultrasound in Pregnancy

I. Ultrasound Features in First Trimester Before 14 Weeks
 A. Week 4: Gestational sac
 B. Week 5–6: Yolk sac
 C. Week 6–7: Fetal pole with heart motion
 D. Week 8: Appearance of midgut herniation (disappears at week 12)
II. Gestational Sac
 A. Mean sac diameter is calculated as the mean of the anteroposterior diameter, the transverse diameter, and the longitudinal diameter.
 B. Gestational age in days = 30 days + mean sac diameter in mm.
III. Crown Rump Length
 A. **Crown rump length** measurement in the first trimester is the best ultrasound method in determination of gestational age.
 B. The average crown rump length from 3 measurements is accurate.
IV. Second and Third Trimesters (After 14 weeks)
 A. Measurements of biparietal diameter, head circumference, abdominal circumference, and femur length before 22 weeks are comparable to crown rump length measurement.

Complicated Obstetrics

Antepartum Testing

Antepartum fetal testing prevents fetal death in high-risk pregnancies. Antepartum testing usually begins at 32–34 weeks.

I. **Indications**
  A. **Maternal Conditions.** Common material indications for antepartum testing include chronic hypertension, gestational hypertension, preeclampsia, diabetes mellitus, gestational diabetes mellitus on medications, systemic lupus erythematosus, renal disease, hemoglobinopathies, cyanotic heart disease, severe asthma, and antiphospholipid syndrome
  B. **Fetal Conditions**: Fetal indications for antepartum testing include prolonged pregnancy, decreased fetal movements, isoimmunization, previous stillbirth, intrauterine growth restriction, oligohydramnios, polyhydramnios, and fetal anomalies.

II. **Techniques**
  A. **Fetal Movement**
    1. Fetal movement counting should start at 32 weeks if medically indicated.
    2. Ten distinct fetal movements in 2 hours are reassuring.
  B. **Fetal Heart Rate Assessment**
    1. Normal fetal heart rate tracing has a baseline of 110–160 bpm, moderate variability, no late or variable decelerations, and accelerations present or absent
  C. **Nonstress Test**
    1. Reactive nonstress test is defined as:
      a) At least 2 accelerations ≥15 bpm, lasting 15 seconds in 20 minute period
      b) Two accelerations ≥10 bpm for 10 seconds in a 20 minute period is reassuring if <32 weeks.
    2. 90% of fetuses have an NST reactive at 32 weeks; 85% at 28 weeks. And 40% at 24 weeks.
    3. A vibroacoustic device can be used to stimulate the fetus if the nonstress test is nonreactive.
  D. **Contraction Stress Test**
    1. Uterine contractions can be induced with nipple stimulation or IV oxytocin. 3 contractions of ≥40 second duration in a 10-minute period is adequate; <3 contractions in 10 min is unsatisfactory.
    2. The contraction stress test is infrequently used.
    3. Interpretation of the contraction stress test:
      a) Negative: no late or significant variable decelerations
      b) Positive: late decelerations with >50% of contractions
      c) Suspicious: inconsistent late decelerations or significant variable decelerations
  E. **Amniotic Fluid Volume Assessment**
    1. Amniotic fluid is composed of fetal urine and fetal lung fluid. The near-term fetus excretes 1,000–1,500 ml of urine per day. Fetal swallowing removes 500–700 ml of amniotic fluid and the intramembranes resorb 420 ml of amniotic fluid per day.
    2. **Clinical Measurement of Amniotic Fluid**
      a) Amniotic fluid index and maximum vertical pocket are frequently used to evaluate the volume of amniotic fluid.

b) Amniotic fluid index is the uterus is divided into 4 quadrants. The vertical diameters of the largest pocket in each quadrant are added together.

c) Maximum vertical is the vertical dimension of the largest fluid pocket.

Antepartum Fetal Surveillence

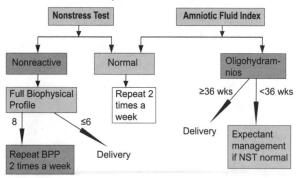

III. Oligohydramnios

A. Oligohydramnios is defined as an amniotic fluid index of ≤5 or MVP of <2. Amniotic fluid index 5–8 cm is borderline. Oligohydramnios and borderline amniotic fluid index at 24–34 weeks are associated with major fetal malformations, intrauterine growth restriction and preterm birth.

B. **Etiology**
   1. Maternal causes of oligohydramnios include dehydration, hypertension, and renal disease
   2. Fetal: renal agenesis, genitourinary tract obstruction, and maternal vascular disease resulting in impaired fetoplacental perfusion.
   3. PPROM, post-term, intrauterine growth restriction, and uteroplacental insufficiency may cause oligohydramnios.

C. **Treatment of Oligohydramnios**. If the mother is dehydrated, give 2L of water orally then reassess amniotic fluid.

IV. Polyhydramnios

A. Polyhydramnios is defined as amniotic fluid index ≥24–25 or MVP >8.

B. Etiologies of polyhydramnios includes fetal upper GI obstruction, anencephaly, genetic disorders, maternal diabetes mellitus, fetal neuromuscular disorder, and idiopathic.

C. **Treatment of Polyhydramnios**
   1. Severe polyhydramnios is treated amnioreduction may be used to decrease maternal discomfort.
   2. Amnioreduction has been associated with rupture of membranes, preterm labor and placenta abruption.

V. Biophysical Profile Scoring

A. Each of five parameters is given a score of 0 or 2.

B. Breathing: at least one episode of ≥ 30 seconds of sustained breathing in 30 min of observation under ultrasound.

C. Gross body movement: ≥ 3 discrete body/limb movements in 30 min

D. Fetal tone: ≥ 1 episode of extension of extremity with return to flexion, or opening or closing of hand.

E. Reactive nonstress test: ≥ 2 accelerations in 30 min

F. AF volume: ≥ 1 pocket of amniotic fluid of ≥ 2 cm or amniotic fluid index ≥ 5.

VI. Modified Biophysical Profile

A. The modified biophysical profile consists of the nonstress test and amniotic fluid index. The MBPP is the most frequently used tool for antenatal testing

B. The nonstress test reflects fetal well-being.

C. The amniotic fluid index is a long-term indicator of uteroplacental function.

VII. Treatment Based on the Biophysical Profile Scores

A. *Score 8–10:* Normal fetus with low risks of chronic asphyxia. Repeat BPP weekly or twice weekly

B. *Score 6:* Consider delivery if ≥ 36 weeks. Deliver if oligohydramnios. If not planning for delivery, deliver if repeat biophysical profile remains ≤ 6; If repeat biophysical profile is more than 6, observe and repeat testing.

C. *Score 4*: Deliver if ≥ 36 weeks. If < 32 weeks, repeat biophysical profile in 4 to 6 hours.

D. *Score 0–2*: Deliver.

VIII. Fetal Lung Maturity Tests

A. Fetal lung maturity can be assumed at 39 weeks of gestation.

B. Perform fetal lung maturity tests on amniotic fluid if planning delivery at <39 weeks. Fetal lung maturity tests are performed after 32 weeks.

IX. Commonly Used Testing Methods

A. Fluorescence polarization with TDx-fetal lung maturity analyzer is positive if ≥ 55. The test is indeterminate if 40–54. The test is immature if ≤ 39.

B. Lecithin/sphingomyelin ratio: positive if ≥2. Blood and meconium can alter the result.

C. Phosphatidylglycerol is positive if present.

Intrauterine Growth Restriction

I. Definition

A. Intrauterine growth restriction is a weight less than the 10th percentile for gestational age.

B. **Severe intrauterine growth restriction** is a weight less than the third percentile. Severe IUGR is associated with adverse perinatal outcomes.

C. **Symmetric intrauterine growth restriction** is caused by early insults. Symmetric IUGR results from aneuploidy, congenital malformation, drugs, and infections. Symmetric IUGR is associated with worse outcome compared to asymmetric IUGR.

D. **Asymmetric intrauterine growth restriction** is usually due to placental and vascular inadequacy in late pregnancy. Asymmetric IUGR has a better prognosis.

II. Etiologies of IUGR

A. Fetal causes of IUGR include chromosomal anomalies, malformations, infections, and multiple gestations.

B. Placental causes of IUGR include small placenta, placental abruption, and previa.

C. Maternal causes of IUGR include hypertension, vascular diseases, infections, thrombophilia, smoking, drug abuse, malnutrition, and high altitude

III. Evaluation and Diagnosis

A. IUGR should be suspected if the fundal height is significantly less than the gestation age. An ultrasound should be performed if the fundal

height is more than 3 cm less than the gestation weeks (30% sensitivity).
B. **Ultrasound**
C. Fetal biometry is diagnostic for IUGR
D. Measurements of abdominal circumference, biparietal diameter, head circumference, and femur length provide most accurate estimate of fetal weight.
E. **Umbilical Artery Doppler Velocimetry** is used for detection of intrauterine growth restriction. Decreased Doppler velocimetry is a sign of placental dysfunction.
F. **Doppler Indices**
   1. Systolic peak velocity/diastolic peak velocity ratio is abnormal if the S/D ratio is greater than 3.0, or if RI is >0.6 at ≥28 weeks.
   2. Absent end-diastolic flow (AEDF) and reversed end-diastolic flow (REDF) are signs of poor fetal condition.
G. **Laboratory Tests for IUGR**
   1. Maternal serum viral screening.
   2. Amniocentesis for fetal karyotyping.
   3. Amniotic fluid PCR for cytomegalovirus and toxoplasmosis.
IV. **Constitutionally Small Fetus**
   A. Normal fetal anatomy, umbilical artery Doppler flow, and amniotic fluid.
   B. Maternal risk factors for intrauterine growth restriction are not present. One or both parents may have been small at birth or of short statue.
   C. No intervention is necessary for constitutionally small fetus.
V. **Treatment**
   A. Uncomplicated singleton intrauterine growth restriction should be delivered at 38–39 weeks.
   B. Deliver is indicated regardless of gestational age if fetal surveillance suggests impending fetal death.
   C. **34–37 Weeks**. Deliver if oligohydramnios, abnormal Doppler studies, maternal risk factors or co-morbidity.
   D. **< 34 Weeks**. Betamethasone is given to promote fetal lung maturity. Perform weekly with umbilical artery Doppler flow, twice weekly biophysical profile, and growth scan every 4 weeks.

Intrauterine Fetal Demise

Intrauterine fetal demise is defined as fetal death after 20 weeks of gestation or of a fetus weighing 350 grams or more. Overall incidence of IUFD is 6.2/1,000 births. Perinatal death is the death of a neonate <28 days of age or fetus >20 weeks.

I. **Conditions Associated with IUFD**
   A. Maternal: hypertension, diabetes mellitus, systemic lupus erythematosus, thyroid disease, renal disease, liver disease, cholestasis, antiphospholipid syndrome, alloimmunization, smoking, obesity, advanced maternal age, and African-American race.
   B. Fetal: congenital malformations, chromosomal anomalies, intrauterine growth restriction, multiple gestations, and fetomaternal hemorrhage
   C. Vasa previa and placental abruption
   D. Umbilical cord: velamentous insertion and cord entanglement
II. **Pathological Findings**
   A. Placenta and cord disease are the main causes of stillbirth (65%). Placental infarction is the single most frequent etiology (18%). Abruption accounts for 7%. Cord complication accounts for 5%.
   B. Other etiologies: fetal anomaly 5.3%. Infection 1.9%. Other 4.8%

C. Unknown etiology: 23.1%.
III. **Evaluation**
   A. Stillbirth should be confirmed with ultrasound.
   B. Disseminated intravascular coagulation in fetal death infrequently occurs.
   C. **Laboratory Studies**
      1. Type and screen, CBC, RPR or VDRL, parvovirus B-19 IgG and IgM, Kleihauer-Betke test, urine drug screen, TSH, lupus anticoagulant, and anticardiolipin antibodies
IV. **Delivery after IUFD**
   A. **Misoprostol for Fetal Demise in Second Trimester**
      1. Vaginal misoprostol: 200–400 µg q4h until delivery of fetus and placenta. Vaginal misoprostol 600 µg single dose has a 73% success rate.
   B. **Fetal Demise in Third Trimester**
      1. Misoprostol start with misoprostol 25–50 µg vaginally and repeat q4h. Double the dose if the first dose is not effective.
      2. Oxytocin: if the cervix is unfavorable, start cervical ripening with misoprostol 25–50 µg vaginally and repeat q4h. Mechanical cervical ripening with Foley catheter may also be used.
   C. **Patients with Previous Cesarean**
      1. In the second trimester, both dilation and evacuation and labor induction with prostaglandins are reasonable options.
      2. After 28 weeks, a Foley catheter balloon should be used for cervical ripening.
   D. **Postpartum Care**
      1. The fetus, placenta, and cord should be examined. Document dysmorphic features and gross abnormalities. The placenta should be sent to pathology.
      2. If postdelivery karyotype is planned, obtain fetal tissues, e.g., placental block (1x1 cm) below the cord insertion site, umbilical cord (1.5 cm), fetal costochondral junction, or patella.

Preterm Labor

Preterm birth is a delivery before completed 37 gestational weeks. Late preterm birth is defined as delivery between 34 0/7 and 36 6/7 weeks. Low birth weight is a neonate less than 2,500 g. Very low birth weight is a neonate weighing less than 1,500 g

I. **Morbidities Related to Preterm Birth**
   A. Neonatal: respiratory distress syndrome, intraventricular hemorrhage, bronchopulmonary dysplasia, patent ductus arteriosus, necrotizing enterocolitis, sepsis, and retinopathy.
   B. Chronic lung diseases, cerebral palsy, vision and hearing impairment, and CNS abnormalities.
   C. NICUs usually provide intensive care at 24 gestational weeks.
II. **Risk Factors for Preterm Birth**
   A. Multiple gestations, previous preterm birth, bleeding after first trimester, and cervical length ≤25 mm ≤24 wks
   B. Bacterial vaginosis is associated with preterm labor; however, antibiotic therapy does not lower the risk of preterm birth.
III. **Prevention of Preterm Labor.** Bed rest, pelvic rest, hydration, tocolytics, and antibiotics are not beneficial.

IV. Cervical Length
A. Short cervical length is ≤25 mm at 14–28 weeks is associated with preterm labor.
B. Cervical length measurement can be measured at 18–22 weeks when performing fetal anatomy survey.
C. **Incidentally Detected Short Cervical Length**
   1. Short cervical length detected by abdominal ultrasound should be confirmed by vaginal ultrasound.
   2. Vaginal progesterone is administered at 24 weeks if cervical length is ≤20 mm at ≤24 weeks.

V. Prevention of Preterm Labor with Progesterone
A. Progesterone reduces the incidence of preterm labor, but there is no improvement in severe intraventricular hemorrhage, NEC, bronchopulmonary dysplasia, or perinatal death.
B. Progesterone is indicated in patients with history of spontaneous preterm birth or a shortened cervix between 10 and 20 mm.
C. **Progesterone Therapy**
   1. 17α-hydroxyprogesterone, 250 mg weekly IM starting at 16–20 weeks
   2. Vaginal progesterone, 90 mg gel (Crinone 8%) daily or vaginal micronized progesterone, 200 mg daily

VI. Evaluation and Diagnosis of Preterm Labor
A. **Speculum Examination**
   1. A speculum examination should always be done before digital examination.
   2. The cervix should be examined for dilation, lesions, or bleeding.
   3. A sample should be obtained from the posterior fornix with a swab for fetal fibronectin.
   4. Collect sample from the lower vagina and rectum or perianal area for group B streptococcus culture.
   5. Collect specimen for wet mount if vaginal infection is suspected.
   6. Gonorrhea and chlamydia testing should be done if the patient is high risk or if no prenatal care
B. **Cervical Examination**
   1. Evaluate for cervical dilation by estimating the size of the internal os.
   2. Multiparous women may have cervical dilation in the third trimester without other preterm labor.
   3. If the patient has vaginal bleeding, perform ultrasound to exclude placenta previa before performing digital exam.
C. **Ultrasound**
   1. Abdominal ultrasound for fetal biometrics, amniotic fluid index, fetal presentation, and location of the placental.
   2. Transvaginal ultrasound for cervical length
      a) Cervical length more than 30 mm indicates that preterm labor unlikely
      b) Cervical length 20–30 mm plus contractions indicates that preterm labor more likely
      c) Cervical length <20 mm plus contractions indicates high risk for preterm labor
G. **Criteria for Preterm Labor Admission**
   1. Persistent and painful contractions at a frequency of 6 or more per hour
   2. Rupture of membranes
   3. Vaginal bleeding
   4. Dilation ≥3 cm and/or effacement ≥80%

H. **Fetal Fibronectin**
   1. Fetal fibronectin has a positive predictive value of less than 20%. Negative predictive value of 69–92%. A negative test excludes the occurance of preterm delivery in the next 1–2 weeks. A positive test is not predictive of preterm labor.
   2. Fetal fibronectin testing is not reliable if the specimen is contaminated with blood, semen, or gel.
   3. The fetal fibronectin test is not needed:
      a) Gestation <24 weeks or ≥34 weeks
      b) Membranes have ruptured
      c) Cervix is dilated more than 3 cm
      d) Intracervical exam or vaginal ultrasound in the last 24 hours

I. **Combination of Cervical Length and Fetal Fibronectin**
   1. Collect fFN sample before vaginal ultrasound
   2. If cervical length is greater than 30 mm, no fetal fibronectin testing is needed
   3. If cervical length is 20 and 30 mm, perform fetal fibronectin testing

VII. **Treatment of Preterm Labor**
   A. Expectant management if ≥34 weeks or <24 weeks.
   B. Administer corticosteroids, group B streptococcus prophylaxis, and tocolysis if between 24 and 34 weeks.
   C. Amniocentesis may be used to confirm fetal lung maturity, karyotype, and infection testing. Amniotic fluid glucose <15 mg/dl and bacteria on Gram stain suggest infection. A positive culture confirms the infection.
   D. Fetal heart rate monitoring is indicted for very preterm fetuses. A nonreassuring fetal heart rate patterns during labor requires cesarean delivery.

VIII. **Antenatal Corticosteroids**
   A. Betamethasone is the most beneficial intervention for enhancing neonatal lung function and reducing the incidence of respiratory distress syndrome, intraventricular hemorrhage, and NEC.
   B. Betamethasone should be given to women at risk of preterm delivery at 24–34 weeks' gestation.
   C. Betamethasone 12 mg IM q 24 hours for 2 doses (or dexamethasone 6 mg IM q 12 hours for 4).

IX. **Group B Streptococcus Prophylaxis**
   A. If no group B streptococcus culture was performed, obtain culture and administer penicillin 5 million units IV, then 2.5–3 million units IV q4h. Discontinue penicillin if group B streptococcus culture result is negative.
   B. If group B streptococcus positive, give penicillin for at least 48 hr.
   C. If group B streptococcus negative, no prophylaxis is given. Culture should be repeated in 5 weeks if not delivered.

X. **Tocolysis and Commonly Used Tocolytic Agents**
   A. Tocolytics may prolong pregnancy for 2 to 7 days to allow maternal administration of betamethasone.
   B. Maintenance tocolysis is not advised.
   C. **Nifedipine**
      1. Used for patients >32 weeks
      2. Protocol: 30 mg PO loading dose, then 10–20 mg q4–6h
      3. Contraindicated in cardiac disease and hypotension
   D. **Magnesium Sulfate**
      1. **Dosage:** 4–6 g IV bolus over a period of 20 min, then 2–3 g IV hourly.
      2. **Contraindicated** in myasthenia gravis.
      3. Magnesium sulfate is used for neuroprotection. Magnesium may reduce the severity and risk of cerebral palsy when given before 32 weeks.

E. **Indomethacin**
   1. Used for patients <32 weeks gestation
   2. 50–100 mg PO or rectally as loading dose, then 25–50 mg PO q6h for 48h.
   3. Contraindicated in renal or hepatic impairment or after 32 weeks. Fetal side effects: constriction of ductus arteriosus, pulmonary hypertension, oligohydramnios, intraventricular hemorrhage, hyperbilirubinemia, and NEC.

F. **Absolute and Relative Contraindications to Tocolytics**
   1. Absolute contraindications include severe preeclampsia, severe placental abruption, severe bleeding, chorioamnionitis, fetal demise, fetal anomaly incompatible with life, and severe IUGR.
   2. Relative contraindications include mild preeclampsia, mild abruption, stable previa, maternal cardiac disease, hyperthyroidism, uncontrolled diabetes, mild intrauterine growth restriction, and cervical dilation >5 cm.

Cervical Insufficiency

Cervical insufficiency is the inability to retain a pregnancy in the absence of contractions.

I. **Clinical Evaluation**
   A. History of ≥ 2 second-trimester pregnancy losses not caused by preterm labor or abruption suggests cervical insufficiency.
   B. Cervical insufficiency causes painless cervical dilation.
   C. Patients often have a history of cervical trauma due to cone biopsy, lacerations, or cervical dilation

II. **Cerclage**
   A. Prophylactic or elective cerclage is accomplished at 13 to 16 weeks after confirming a live fetus with no anomalies. Urgent or emergent cerclage is done at 16 to 24 after cervical dilation has already occurred.
   B. Cerclage is contraindicated if contractions, placental abruption, or chorioamnionitis are present.
   C. Cerclage is not effective in reducing preterm delivery in low-risk women with incidental cervical shortening (≤15 mm).
   D. Cerclage in twin gestations results in a higher rate of preterm birth.

III. **Indications for Cerclage**
   A. If there is history of cervical insufficiency, the cerclage should be placed at 13 to 15 weeks.
   B. Singleton pregnancy with cervical length <25 mm at 15 to 23 weeks and a history of preterm birth <34 weeks.

IV. **Cerclage Techniques**
   A. Most cerclages are done vaginally with the McDonald technique. Place Mersilene tape or Prolene suture in a purse-string fashion high at cervicovaginal junction.
   B. Tie the knot and leave a long end for future removal.

Preterm Premature Rupture of Membranes

I. **Definition, Etiology and Epidemiology**
   A. Preterm premature rupture of membrane is defined as rupture of membrane before 37 weeks of gestation. After 37 weeks, membrane rupture before onset of regular contractions is called premature rupture of membranes (PROM).

B. The cause of spontaneous PPROM is usually not known. Risk factors for PPROM including intrauterine infection, placenta abruption, previous premature rupture of membranes, and smoking.

C. PPROM causes 30% of preterm births.

II. Clinical Manifestations

A. PPROM presents with a sudden gush of fluid from vagina, followed by uterine contractions.

B. PPROM may also present as intermittent leaking of fluid from vagina.

III. Speculum Examination and Testing

A. Inspect the cervix and assess for amniotic fluid pooling. Visualization of fluid flowing from cervical os or pooling of amniotic fluid is diagnostic of rupture of membranes.

B. Fern test provides indirect evidence for rupture of membranes, but not completely reliable. Dry amniotic fluid demonstrates a fernlike pattern under microscope.

C. Collect amniotic fluid for fetal lung maturity testing if >32 weeks.

D. Collect sample for group B streptococcus culture.

E. Do not perform digital cervical exam because of risk of infection.

IV. AmniSure Test

A. The AmniSure test detects placental α-microgobulin-1 (PAMG-1), which is an amniotic fluid protein.

B. 97.2% positive agreement and 97.6% negative agreement with diagnosis.

C. A false-positive AmniSure result may be caused by vaginal bleeding.

V. Amniocentesis and Instillation of Indigo Carmine

A. Indigo-carmine instillation is used in ambiguous cases. Instill 1 ml of indigo carmine in 9 ml of NS.

B. Rupture of membranes is confirmed if a vaginal tampon is stained with the blue dye.

VI. Ultrasound

A. Oligohydramnios is suggestive of rupture of membranes, but is not diagnostic.

VII. Treatment

A. Admit to labor and delivery and start electronic fetal monitoring.

B. Observe for signs of labor, chorioamnionitis (fever ≥38.0° C) and placental abruption (bleeding and pain).

C. Delivery is indicated if intrauterine infection is present or if nonreassuring fetal heart rate pattern develops.

D. Prolonging the pregnancy after rupture of membranes is associated with intrauterine infection and neonatal sepsis.

VIII. Treatment Based on Gestational Age

A. **≥ 34 Weeks.** Delivery is indicated.

B. **32–34 Weeks**
   1. Deliver if fetal lung maturity is confirmed.
   2. Expectant management if fetal lung maturity is negative.
   3. Administer steroids for fetal lung maturity and antibiotics to prolong the latency.

C. **24–32 Weeks**
   1. Accelerate fetal lung maturity with betamethasone, 12 mg IM every 24 hours for 2 doses
   2. Antibiotic prophylaxis to prolong latency (7-day antibiotic regimen):
      a) Ampicillin 2 g plus erythromycin 250 mg IV q6h for 48 hours. Followed by amoxicillin 250 mg plus enteric-coated erythromycin-base 333 mg po q8h for 5 days.
      b) Alternative: Azithromycin (Zithromax) 1g PO and ampicillin 2 g IV q6h for 48h, then amoxicillin 500 mg PO tid or 875 mg PO 2 times a day for 5 days.

   D. **<23–24 Weeks**: Expectant management. No need for group B strepto-
      coccus prophylaxis, antibiotics or steroids.
IX. **Group B Streptococcus Prophylaxis**
   A. Continue antibiotics for group B streptococcus prophylaxis for 48 hours.
   B. No additional antibiotics should be given if the patient receiving ampicil-
      lin.
X. **Tocolytics** are not effective in the setting of rupture of membranes.
XI. **Antepartum Care**
   A. PPROM before 23 weeks can be discharged home for expectant man-
      agement, then readmit at 24 weeks for steroids and antibiotics.

Placental Abruption

I. **Risk Factors**
   A. Risk factors for placental abruption include trauma, prior abruption, co-
      caine abuse, hypertension, preeclampsia, smoking, preterm labor and
      premature rupture of membranes, advanced maternal age, uterine
      anomaly, and multiparity
   B. Subchorionic hemorrhage on ultrasound in first or second trimester is
      associated with placental abruption, early and late pregnancy loss, pre-
      term labor, and PPROM.

Visible Bleeding

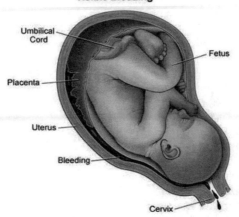

I. **Diagnosis**
   A. Abruption is diagnosed by the findings of abdominal pain and vaginal
      bleeding in the third trimester.
   B. Mild abruption can be asymptomatic. Severe abruption can cause fetal
      death and disseminated intravascular coagulation.
   C. Electronic fetal monitoring demonstrates frequent uterine contractions
      and variable or late decelerations, decreased variability, or bradycardia

D. **Ultrasound**
   1. Ultrasound is not sensitive for placenta abruption unless the abruption is severe. Ultrasound is useful to exclude placenta previa.
   2. Abruption may appear on ultrasound as a thickened placenta. Acute bleeding is hyperechoic. Hematoma or clot becomes isoechoic at 3 days. A hypoechoic area seen at 1–2 weeks.

II. **Laboratory Studies**
   A. CBC, type and screen, INR, partial thromboplastin time, and fibrinogen
   B. Most abruptions are associated with normal lab values.
   C. **Calculation of Fetomaternal Hemorrhage**
      1. The Kleihauer-Betke test measures fetal red blood cells in maternal circulation. The Kleihauer Betke test is used to calculate the dosage of RhIG for a Rh-negative patient. The KB test has some value in the diagnosis of abruption.
      2. Flow cytometry is a more accurate assay for fetal red blood cells in the maternal circulation.
      3. The simple formula for estimation of fetal blood in the maternal circulation = mL of fetal blood = % of fetal blood cell on KB for 5,000. For example: 2% of fetal blood cells on a Kleihauer-Betke test means 100 ml (0.02 for 5,000 ml) of fetal whole blood in maternal circulation, and 4 vials of RhIG is required in a Rh-negative patient. The simple formula overestimates FMH.
      4. Formula: 5000 for maternal hematocrit for % fetal cells in KB/0.5

III. **Treatment**
   A. **Term or Near Term (>37 Weeks)**
      1. Delivery: vaginal delivery is preferred if maternal and fetal status is reassuring.
   B. **Preterm with Reassuring Maternal and Fetal Status**
      1. **34–37 Weeks:** Perform amniocentesis and deliver if fetal lung maturity test is positive.
      2. **24–34 Weeks**: Expectant management with close monitoring, serial ultrasound, betamethasone, and group B streptococcus prophylaxis. Tocolysis with magnesium sulfate is not contraindicated.
   C. **Severe Abruption with Nonreassuring Maternofetal Status**
   D. **≥24 Weeks:** Deliver
   E. **<24 Weeks**: Maternal resuscitation and delivery

Placenta Previa

I. **Terminology**
   A. Placenta previa is a placenta covering internal os (partial or complete previa). Low-lying placenta is when the edge of placenta is 1 mm to 20 mm from the internal os. In second trimester, the placenta should normally be more than 20 cm from the internal os.
   B. **Complete previa** is when the placenta completely covers internal os.
   C. **Partial previa** is when the placenta partially covers internal os.
   D. **Marginal Previa** is when the edge of the placenta is ≤2 cm from the internal os.
   E. **Low-lying placenta** is when placenta is implanted in the lower uterine segment and the edge is >2 cm from the internal os.
   F. **Placenta accreta** is when the placenta invades into the uterus, resulting in abnormal adherence of the placenta to the uterus.
   G. **Placenta increta** is when the placenta invades the myometrium.
   H. **Placenta Percreta occurs when the** placenta invades through myometrium and serosa.

I. **Vasa Previa** occurs when the fetal blood vessels running through placental membrane cross over the cervix unprotected. Vessel rupture in labor causes rapid fetal exsanguination.

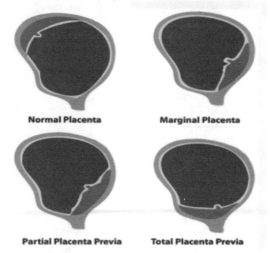

Normal Placenta   **Marginal Placenta**

Partial Placenta Previa   **Total Placenta Previa**

Figure: Types of placenta previa

II. **Risk Factors for Placenta Previa**
 A. Prior cesarean, uterine curettage, advanced maternal age, and multiparity

III. **Diagnosis**
 A. Placenta previa presents with painless vaginal bleeding in the third trimester. Contractions may sometimes occur with bleeding.
 B. Placenta previa is usually diagnosed in early pregnancy by ultrasound. Intracervical exam should not be performed if placenta previa is suspected.
 C. 90% of placenta previa diagnosed before 20 weeks will resolve spontaneously by term. A repeat scan at 28–32 weeks is advised.
 D. Endovaginal ultrasound is diagnostic for placental previa.

IV. **Treatment**
 A. Complete and partial previa requires cesarean delivery.
 B. Outpatient management of asymptomatic previa: Ultrasound q2–4 weeks and avoidance of intercourse and exercise.
 C. **Timing of Cesarean Delivery**
  1. Placenta previa should be delivered at 36–37 weeks.
  2. Amniocentesis for fetal lung maturity is not required.
 D. **Marginal Previa or Low-lying Placenta**
  1. If the lower edge of placenta is more than 20 mm from the internal os, labor is managed as a normal pregnancy.
  2. Vaginal delivery is recommended if the placenta is 10 to 20 mm from the internal os. The antepartum bleeding risk is 3%.
  3. If the lower edge of placenta is within 10 mm of the internal os, cesarean delivery is advised due to the high risk of bleeding.

E. **Placenta Previa with Acute Bleeding**
   1. Laboratory Studies: CBC, type and screen, coagulation panel. Maintain the hematocrit >30
   2. **If ≥ 36 Weeks**: Perform cesarean delivery
   3. **If < 36 Weeks**
      a) Expectant management
      b) Deliver if severe hemorrhage
      c) Give betamethasone between 24 to 34 weeks. Tocolysis is acceptable if patient has contractions
      d) Criteria for discharge: The patient must be asymptomatic, bleeding-free for 48 hours, hematocrit >30%, vitals within normal limits, and rapid access to the hospital. Intercourse should be avoided.
F. **Placenta Previa with Accreta**. Delivery at 34–35 weeks of gestational age before labor begins and hemorrhage occurs.
G. **Cesarean Hysterectomy**
   1. Cesarean hysterectomy is frequently advised if the patient desires no future fertility.
   2. Make the uterine incision away from placenta. Close the uterine incision after delivery of the fetus and then proceed with hysterectomy.
H. **Uterine Preservation**
   1. Uterine preservation is associated with hemorrhage and infection.
   2. Fecal placenta accreta may be removed manually with oversewing of the bleeding sites.
   3. If the placenta cannot be removed, the placenta may be left in situ. Uterine conservation occurs in 78%.

Multiple Gestation

I. **Complications Associated with Multiple Gestation**
   A. Multiple gestations are associated with preterm delivery, intrauterine growth restriction, congenital anomalies, malpresentation, fetal death, cord entanglement, placenta previa, placental abruption, preeclampsia, gestational diabetes, and postpartum hemorrhage
II. **Dizygotic Twins**
   A. Dizygotic twins originate from 2 separate ova, are genetically different, and have separate placentae and membranes
   B. Different sex of fetus rules out monozygotic twins
   C. 20% multiple gestations in in-vitro fertilization patients are twins
   D. **Monozygotic twins** occur when 1 fertilized ovum splits in 2. Monozygotic twins are the same sex and are genetically identical.
III. **Ultrasound Features of Chorionicity and Amnionicity**
   A. Monochorionicity occurs in 20% of twins and is associated with complications.
IV. **Treatment of Twin Gestations**
   A. **Antepartum Care**
      1. Ultrasound every 2–6 weeks in second or third trimester to screen for fetal growth restriction. Monochorionic twins need an ultrasound every 2 weeks.
      2. Cervical length is associated with an increased risk of preterm labor if cervical length ≤25 mm at 24–26 weeks.
      3. Antenatal testing should start at 32 weeks if monochorionic or if >20% growth discordance

B. **Growth Discordance**
   1. Calculated by EFW of larger twin (grams) – EFW of smaller twin (grams) / EFW of the larger twin (grams). ≥20% is defined as discordance.
C. **Timing of Delivery**
   1. Uncomplicated dichorionic twins should be delivered at 38 weeks.
   2. Uncomplicated diamniotic-monochorionic twins are delivered at 34–37 weeks.
   3. Monoamniotic twins should be delivered at 32–34 weeks
D. **Route of Delivery**
   1. Second twins have worse prognosis than first twins. Cesarean rate for twins is 75%.
   2. Vertex/vertex (40%)—vaginal delivery
   3. Vertex/breech (40%)—vaginal delivery
   4. Presenting twin non-vertex (20%)—cesarean section
E. **Vaginal Delivery of Twins**
   1. Deliver twins in the operating room with ultrasound available.
   2. Two approaches for vaginal delivery of nonvertex second twin:
   3. Breech extraction of second twin if EFW is >2,000 grams
   4. External cephalic version of second twin after the first is delivered

Alloimmunization

Alloimmunization is the development of maternal antibodies against fetal antigens on the RBC membranes, resulting in fetal hemolysis, anemia, heart failure, hydrops, and hyperbilirubinemia.

I. **RhD Alloimmunization**
   A. Rh+ is D positive in 87% in Caucasians, 93% in African Americans, 99% in Native Americans and Asians
II. **Prevention of Alloimmunization in RhD-Negative Women**
   A. Determine the paternal Rh status. If negative, no further therapy is needed.
   B. Give RhIG 300 µg IM at 28 weeks of gestation. RhIG will not be effective if alloimmunization has already occurred (positive anti-D antibody). Antibody screen should be obtained prior to administering RhIG to diagnose pre-existing sensitization.
   C. At birth, newborn Rh status is assessed by cord blood typing. If negative, no further therapy. If positive, give mother 300 µg RhIG to protect against sensitization by 30 ml of fetal whole blood. RhIG should be given within 72 hours postpartum.
   D. The rosette test may be performed at the time of delivery to screen for excessive fetomaternal hemorrhage (FMH). If rosette test is positive, perform Kleihauer-Betke (KB) stain or fetal cell stain with flow cytometry.
III. **Treatment of First Sensitized Pregnancy**
   A. Assess antibody titer if antibody screen has a positive anti-D antibody.
   B. Critical titer values are usually between 8 and 16. Critical titer for anti-Kell is 1:8, and for all other antibodies 1:16.
   C. **If paternal RhD-negative**: Only surveillance is needed
   D. **If paternal RhD-positive**
      1. Consider determining fetal Rh status by amniocentesis or fetal DNA testing using maternal plasma. RhD-negative fetus needs routine care only, but repeat titer in 4–6 weeks to exclude error in fetal testing.

2. If fetal RhD-positive, assess titer every 4 weeks. Once titer is ≥16, obtain middle cerebral artery peak systolic velocity every 1–2 weeks from 20 to 34 weeks. If peak systolic velocity is ≥1.5 MoMs, repeat in 2–3 days. Perform cordocentesis and transfusion if values are rising.
3. Start antenatal testing at 32 weeks. Perform amniocentesis for fetal lung maturity at 35 weeks and deliver when lungs are mature.
4. Middle cerebral artery Doppler has superior sensitivity, specificity, and accuracy compared to amniocentesis.
5. Do not give RhIG to sensitized patients. RhIG is not effective for sensitized patients, and interferes with the measurement of endogenously generated anti-D titer.

E. **Subsequently Affected Pregnancies**
  1. Fetal anemia is usually more severe than in first pregnancy. Early amniocentesis is performed to assess fetal Rh status.
  2. Perform early serial amniocentesis and middle cerebral artery Doppler at 18 weeks, repeat every 1–2 weeks.
  3. Maternal titers do not correlate with the severity of fetal anemia.

F. **Non-RhD Antibodies**
  1. Kell alloimmunization is the most common cause of fetal hemolytic anemia. Anti-Kell can rarely cause erythroblastosis fetalis by suppressing erythropoiesis. Amniocentesis is of no value in managing these patients.
  2. Lewis antibodies are IgM and cannot pass through the placenta. Lewis antibody are not harmful to fetus.
  3. Duffy antigens (Fya and Fyb) are common in African Americans. Fya is immunogenic. Fyb is a poor immunogen. Anti-Fya causes fetal hemolytic anemia.
  4. Other atypical antibodies include Lutheran, MNS, I, P, Kidd, and MSSS.
  5. Blood transfusion is the most frequent cause of isoimmunization.
  6. Isoimmunization due to atypical antibodies has the same treatment as RhD isoimmunization.

G. **Hydrops Fetalis**
  1. **Ultrasound Diagnosis**
    a) Hydrops fetalis is skin edema, pericardial effusion, pleural effusion, and ascites.
    b) Hydrops fetalis is associated with polyhydramnios, placental thickening, cardiomegaly, hepato-splenomegaly, and edema of abdominal wall.
  2. **Isoimmune Type hydrops fetalis** is associated with severe fetal anemia and occurs after an intrauterine transfusion or delivery.

3. **Non-immune Type**
   a) Non-immune type hydrops is caused by cardiovascular, chromo-somal and non-chromosomal abnormalities, twin-twin transfusion syndrome, maternal-fetal infections, congenital malformation, anemia, or idiopathic.
   b) Early delivery is unlikely to improve the poor outcome because the survival rate is <20%.

Preeclampsia and Hypertension

Risk factors for hypertension include nulliparity (3% occurrence), multiple gestations, history of preeclampsia, chronic hypertension, diabetes mellitus, gestational diabetes mellitus, renal disease, thrombophilias, African-American race, extremes of maternal age, and obesity.

I. **Diagnostic Criteria**
   A. **Gestational Hypertension**
      1. Blood pressure ≥140/90 mm Hg for the first time during pregnancy and no proteinuria. Blood pressure should be elevated on ≥ two oc-casions, at least 4h apart, and within a 1 week period.
      2. Gestational hypertension usually begins in third trimester and may progress to preeclampsia.
      3. Blood pressure should usually return to normal before 12 weeks postpartum. If hypertension still persists at 12 weeks postpartum, chronic hypertension is diagnosed.
   B. **Criteria for Preeclampsia**
      1. Systolic blood pressure ≥140 or diastolic blood pressure ≥90 mm Hg that occurs after 20 weeks' gestation in a women with previously normal blood pressure. Blood pressure should be elevated on ≥ two occasions, at least 4h apart, and within a 1-week period.
      2. Proteinuria ≥300 mg/24 hours (urine protein 30 mg/dl or ≥1+ on urine dipstick)
   C. **Severe Preeclampsia (if one or more of the following is present)**
      1. Systolic blood pressure ≥160 mm Hg or diastolic blood pressure ≥110 mm Hg on two occasions at least 6 hours apart while the patient is on bed rest
      2. Proteinuria ≥5 g in a 24-hour urine specimen or 3+ or greater on two random urine samples collected at least 4 hours apart
      3. Oliguria of less than 500 ml in 24 hours
      4. Cerebral or visual disturbances
      5. Pulmonary edema or cyanosis
      6. Epigastric or right upper-quadrant pain
      7. Impaired liver function
      8. Thrombocytopenia
      9. Fetal growth restriction
   D. **Eclampsia** is a seizure that cannot be attributed to another etiology in a women with preeclampsia
   E. **Chronic Hypertension**
      1. Blood pressure ≥140/90 mm Hg before pregnancy or diagnosed be-fore 20 weeks' gestation not due to gestational trophoblastic disease OR
      2. Hypertension first diagnosed after 20 weeks' gestation and persistent after 12 weeks' postpartum
   F. **Preeclampsia Superimposed on Chronic hypertension**
      1. One or more of the following is present in patient with chronic hyper-tension:

a) New-onset proteinuria (300 mg/24h) in a women with hypertension and no proteinuria early in pregnancy (<20 weeks)
b) Sudden increase in proteinuria
c) Sudden increase in blood pressure in a woman with previously well controlled hypertension
d) Thrombocytopenia (platelets <100,000/mm^3)
e) Abnormal increase in ALT or AST

II. Treatment of Preeclampsia

A. Mild Gestational Hypertension or Preeclampsia

1. **Initial Evaluation of Hypertension or Preeclampsia**
   a) Evaluate for severe headache, visual changes, epigastric pain, or difficulty breathing.
   b) Assess serial blood pressures and edema.
   c) Laboratory Studies: 24h urine protein, CBC, liver enzymes, and creatinine. Hyperuricemia is associated with renal impairment.
   d) Fetal assessment includes nonstress test, fetal biometry, and amniotic fluid index.

2. **Criteria for Outpatient Treatment**
   a) No symptoms of severe preeclampsia
   b) Gestational age between 32 to 37 weeks
   c) Systolic blood pressure ≤150 and diastolic blood pressure ≤100 mm Hg
   d) Urine protein ≤1,000 mg/24h, normal liver enzymes and platelet count

3. **Outpatient Treatment**
   a) Rest, daily blood pressure and urine dip stick. Daily fetal movement count.
   b) Twice weekly clinic visit, laboratory testing, nonstress test, and amniotic fluid index at each visit
   c) Fetal growth ultrasound and Doppler

4. **Delivery**
   a) Delivery is usually indicated if >37 weeks.
   b) For mild gestational hypertension, MgSO$_4$ is not required during labor and postpartum. For mild preeclampsia, MgSO$_4$ should be given for seizure prophylaxis.

B. Severe Preeclampsia

1. Delivery if accomplished at ≥34 weeks.
2. Keep systolic blood pressure at 140–160 and diastolic blood pressure at 90–100 mm Hg.
3. Give MgSO$_4$ for seizure prophylaxis for 24h.

C. Acute-Onset Hypertension with Systolic ≥160 or Diastolic ≥110

1. Labetalol: 20 mg IV over 2 min. Assess blood pressure in 10 min. If not effective, give 40 mg and assess blood pressure in 10 min. Increase to 80 mg if blood pressure remains >160 mm/Hg. If labetalol fails, give hydralazine 10 mg IV over 2 min.
2. Hydralazine: 5 or 10 mg IV over 2 min and assess blood pressure in 20 min. If not effective, give 10 mg and repeat blood pressure in 20 min. Increase to 20 mg and assess blood pressure in 10 min.
3. Second-line therapy includes labetalol or nicardipine infusion pump. Sodium nitroprusside is used for extreme emergencies.

D. Intrapartum Treatment

1. Epidural anesthesia is preferred for pain (if platelets ≥100,000/µl).
2. Monitor for placenta abruption.
3. Continue magnesium sulfate throughout labor until 24 hr after delivery.

E. **Treatment of Postpartum Hypertension**
   1. For severe hypertension, use the intrapartum regimens for rapid control. Start oral medications if systolic blood pressure is >150 mmHg and/or diastolic blood pressure >100 mmHg.
   2. Nifedipine 10–20 mg every 4–6 hours or nifedipine XL 10–30 mg PO q12h. Labetalol 200–400 mg PO q8–12h
   3. Use ACE inhibitors in patients with diabetes or cardiomyopathy and diuretics in patients with circulatory overload or pulmonary edema. Furosemide 20 mg IV or PO 2 times a day and Hydrochlorothiazide 25–50 mg PO once a day.

HELLP Syndrome

I. **Criteria for HELLP Syndrome**
   A. **H**emolysis: 1) abnormal peripheral smear (schistocytes, burr cells, echinocytes); 2) serum bilirubin >1.2 mg/dl; 3) LDH >600 IU/L
   B. **E**levated **L**iver enzymes: AST ≥72 IU/L; LDH ≥600 IU/L
   C. **L**ow **P**latelets: <100,000/mm^3
II. **Treatment**
   A. Immediate delivery is indicated for disseminated intravascular coagulation, renal failure, abruption, respiratory distress, or liver hematoma
   B. Give steroids if between 24–34 weeks with stable maternal and fetal condition. Then deliver within 24 hours of last dose of dexamethasone.
   C. **Dexamethasone Rescue Protocols**
      1. Dexamethasone 12 mg IM repeat in 12 h
      2. Dexamethasone 6 mg IM q6h for 4 doses
      3. Dexamethasone 10 mg IV q12 h for 2 doses followed by 5 mg IV q12 h for 2 doses or
      4. Dexamethasone 10 mg q12h IV until delivery and 10 mg IV q12h for 3 doses postpartum

Eclampsia

53% of seizures occur antepartum and 11% postpartum (>90% within 1 week after delivery). Seizures may manifest as facial twitching to generalized muscular contractions. Headache and visual disturbance often occur before an eclamptic seizure.

I. **Airway and General Measures:**
   A. Place patient in the lateral decubitus position. Suctions of vomitus and oral secretions. Prevent injury.
   B. Call anesthesia for intubation in status eclampticus; O_2 8–10 L/min by face mask, pulse oximetry, and ABG.
II. **Blood Pressure:**
   A. Administer labetalol or hydralazine to maintain systolic blood pressure at 140–160 mm Hg and diastolic blood pressure 90–110 mm Hg.
III. **Convulsion:**
   A. MgSO$_4$ 6 g IV loading dose then 2–3 g/hr maintenance infusion. Given an additional 2 g IV If convulsion persists or recurs. Administer lorazepam (Ativan) 1–2 mg IV if MgSO$_4$ fails.

Chronic Hypertension

Maternal effects of hypertension includes cardiovascular accidents, pulmonary edema, renal failure, and cardiac decompensation because of increased volume and decreased colloid oncotic pressure. Fetal effects of hypertension include preterm birth, growth restriction, fetal death, placental abruption, and cesarean

I. **Preconceptional and Prenatal Care**
   A. Avoid ACE inhibitors and angiotensin II receptor blockers because of teratogenicity. Patients using ACE inhibitors or ARBs should use contraception. Atenolol causes fetal growth restriction.
   B. Evaluate creatinine, BUN, 24h urinary protein, spot urine protein/creatinine ratio, and creatinine clearance, ECG, echocardiogram, and ophthalmologic evaluation.
   C. Evaluate for secondary causes with severe hypertension: pheochromocytoma, Cushing disease, renal artery stenosis, or primary aldosteronism.
   D. Laboratory Studies: CBC, metabolic panel, and 24hr urine protein every trimester.
   E. Ultrasound at 18–20 weeks. Growth scan q4h after 24 weeks. Twice weekly fetal testing starting at 32 weeks or earlier for severe cases.

II. **Mild hypertension**
   A. Defined as systolic 140–159 mmHg or diastolic 90–109 mm Hg.
   B. Patients with end-organ damage, need to maintain blood pressure in the normal range.

III. **Severe hypertension**
   A. Systolic ≥160 or diastolic ≥110 mm Hg.
   B. Methyldopa 250 mg 3 times a day, up to 4 grams/day
   C. Labetalol 100 mg q8–12h, up to 2,400 mg/day
   D. Nifedipine 10–20 mg 3 times a day or nifedipine XL 30 mg once a day, up to 120 mg/day.

IV. **Delivery**
   A. Earlier delivery is indicated if severe preeclampsia develops or maternal-fetal condition is compromised.

V. **Mild Chronic hypertension**
   A. Vaginal delivery at term is advised for mild hypertension.
   B. Uncomplicated hypertension with no medication at 38–39 week. Hypertension on medication, deliver should be delivered at 37–39 weeks.

Diabetes and Pregnancy

I. **ADA Diagnostic Criteria for Diabetes**
   A. A1C ≥6.5% or
   B. Fasting plasma glucose ≥126/dl or
   C. 2-h plasma glucose ≥200 mg/dl after 75 g glucose or
   D. Random plasma glucose ≥200 mg/dl in a patient with symptoms of hyperglycemia.

II. **Prediabetes**
   A. Impaired fasting glucose: 100–125 mg/dl
   B. Impaired glucose tolerance: 75-g 2-h plasma glucose of 140–199 mg/dl
   C. A1c 5.7–6.4%

III. **Screening for Gestational Diabetes Mellitus**
   A. At first prenatal visit, measure fasting glucose, hemoglobin A1C, or random plasma glucose.
   B. All women not known to have diabetes should undergo a 75-g OGTT at 24–28 weeks. Perform OGTT after an overnight fast of at least 8 hours.
   C. One abnormal value is adequate to make the diagnosis.

IV. ADA Diagnostic Criteria for gestational diabetes mellitus
A. *2-h 75-g Oral Glucose Tolerance Test*
1. Fasting venous plasma glucose: ≥92 but <126 mg/dl
2. 1-hour glucose: ≥180 mg/dl
3. 2-hour glucose: ≥153 mg/dl

V. ADA Diagnostic Criteria for Overt diabetes mellitus
A. Fasting venous plasma glucose: ≥126 mg/dl
B. Hemoglobin A1C: ≥6.5%
C. Random plasma glucose: ≥200 mg/dl

VI. Gestational Diabetes
A. Impaired glucose tolerance first recognized during pregnancy.
B. Pregnancy-related hormonal changes may reveal a genetic susceptibility to type 2 diabetes mellitus. 50% of patients with gestational diabetes mellitus will become diabetic within 15 years.
C. Diabetes is associated with fetal macrosomia, shoulder dystocia, and neonatal complications. Increased risk of stillbirth.

VII. Diet Therapy
A. Nutritional counseling by a registered dietitian. The patient should increase whole grain cereals and complex carbohydrates. The patient should decrease simple sugars and increase fruits and vegetables. Initiate diet therapy (1,800 to 2,500 kcal/day) for 1–2 weeks. If unable to maintain glucose levels in the target range, start medications.
B. Glucose self-monitoring: at least 4 times a day including morning fasting and 2–hour postprandial.

VIII. Target Maternal Capillary Glucose Levels
A. Fasting: <95 mg/dl
B. 1-h postprandial: <140 mg/dl
C. 2-h postprandial: <120 mg/dl

IX. Insulin Therapy
A. **Initial Insulin Dosing with NPH and Regular Insulin Based on Gestational Weeks**
1. <18 weeks: 0.7 unit/kg
2. 18–26 weeks: 0.8 unit/kg
3. 26–36 weeks: 0.9 unit/kg
4. >36 weeks: 1.0 unit/kg

B. **Insulin administration:**
1. Give 2/3 of total daily dose before breakfast and 1/3 at night with the short-acting insulin before dinner and the NPH before bedtime
2. 3-injection regimen:
3. AM dose (2/3 of total daily dose): 2/3 NPH and 1/3 regular insulin before breakfast
4. PM dose (1/3 of total daily dose): 1/2 regular insulin before dinner; 1/2 NPH before bed time
5. Adjust insulin doses and timing every 3–7 days based on patient's response.

C. *Short Acting Insulin*
1. Lispro insulin (Humalog): onset 0.25 hours, peak 0.5–1.5 hours, duration 4–5 hours
2. Aspart insulin (Novolog): onset 0.25 hours, peak 1–3 hours, duration 3–5 hours
3. Regular insulin (Humulin R, Novolin R): onset 0.5 hours, peak 2–5 hours, duration 5–8 hours

D. *Intermediate Acting Insulin*
1. Humulin NPH, Humulin Lente: onset 1–3 hours, peak 6–12 hours, duration 18–24 hours
2. Novolin N: onset 1.5 hours, peak 4–20 hours, duration 24 hours
3. Novolin L: onset 2.5 hours, peak 7–15 hours, duration 22 hours

X. **Oral Hypoglycemics**
  A. **Glyburide**
    1. Glyburide is second generation of sulfonylurea, which stimulates insulin release from pancreatic β cells.
    2. Glyburide crosses placenta. Fetal glyburide level is 70% of maternal level.
    3. Regimen: Start with 2.5 mg AM. Increase AM dose by 2.5 mg every 3–7 days as needed. Add 5 mg PM. Increase AM or PM dose by 5 mg as needed. Max 10 mg 2 times a day.
    4. If glyburide is not successful, add NPH insulin at bed time.
  B. **Metformin**
    1. Metformin is a biguanide, which crosses the placenta. Metformin enhances insulin action on the liver and muscle. Metformin reduces gluconeogenesis. Metformin does not cause hypoglycemia or weight gain; 20% have nausea, abdominal discomfort, and diarrhea.
    2. Metformin is an effective alternative to glyburide or insulin. Metformin may be combined with insulin.
    3. Failure rate of metformin is 35%, compared with glyburide 16%.
    4. Start with 500 mg qd and increase weekly to maximum 2,500 mg daily.

XI. **Antenatal Surveillance and Delivery**
  A. Diet-controlled gestational diabetes mellitus is managed as normal pregnancy. Daily fetal movement counting is started in third trimester. Begin twice weekly nonstress test and amniotic fluid index after 40 weeks. Spontaneous vaginal deliver at term is preferred.
  B. Insulin or oral hypoglycemic-controlled gestational diabetes mellitus is managed with antenatal testing at 32 weeks. Early delivery is not indicated unless the pregnancy is complicated by intrauterine growth restriction or preeclampsia.
  C. If glucose is poorly controlled with medications, consider early delivery at 34–39 weeks.
  D. Macrosomia: Ultrasound is no more accurate than clinical exam in estimating fetal weight in late gestation. Elective cesarean delivery if EFW >4,500g to prevent shoulder dystocia.

XII. **Postpartum Evaluation**
  A. No need to continue antidiabetic drugs postpartum because glucose usually returns to normal.
  B. Check hemoglobin A1c at 6–12 weeks after delivery using nonpregnant criteria and diabetes mellitus screening at least every 3 years.

XIII. **Pregestational Diabetes**
  A. **Complications**
    1. Obstetrical: Increased risk of preeclampsia and cesarean delivery
    2. Fetal effects of diabetes include caudal regression syndrome, neural tube defects, heart defects, renal anomalies, abortion, preterm birth, macrosomia, intrauterine growth restriction, intrauterine fetal demise, and hydramnios
    3. Neonatal effects of diabetes include respiratory distress, hypoglycemia, hyperbilirubinemia, and hypocalcemia
  B. **Preconception Care**
    1. Hemoglobin A1C, 24 urine protein and creatinine, TSH, T4, ECG, and dilated eye exam by an ophthalmologist
    2. Keep blood pressure <130/80 mmHg. Discontinue statins, ACE inhibitors, and ARBs. Use labetalol or nifedipine for hypertension.
    3. Start insulin therapy before pregnancy to lower the hemoglobin A1C to <6% for 3 months before conception.
    4. One mg of folic acid qd for 3 months prior to conception

    C. Prenatal Care
        1. First and Second Trimesters
           a) Clinic visits every 1–2 weeks for glucose control
           b) Perform an early ultrasound for dating. Perform a target ultrasound at 18–20 weeks. Fetal echocardiogram is done at 20–22 weeks. Baseline fetal growth evaluation at 24 weeks
           c) First trimester screening or quadruple screening at 16–18 weeks
        2. Third Trimester
           a) Weekly clinic visit after 28 weeks and fetal movement counting.
           b) Twice weekly nonstress test and amniotic fluid index, starting at 32 weeks.
           c) Repeat fetal growth ultrasound every 4 weeks in the third trimester.
           d) For well controlled diabetes mellitus, early delivery is not required.
           e) If diabetes mellitus poorly controlled, deliver at 34–39 weeks.
    D. Intrapartum Glucose Management
        1. Hold AM insulin.
        2. Maintain glucose level at 70–110 mg/dl.
        3. Assess glucose every 2 hours in latent labor phase and every hour in active phase.
        4. If indicated, cesarean should be scheduled in early morning.
    E. Fluid and Insulin Management
        1. Gestational diabetes mellitus or mild gestational diabetes mellitus, start IV infusion of normal saline at 125 ml/hr. Change to 5% dextrose if glucose <70 mg/dl. Give insulin if glucose is >120 mg/dl. OR
        2. Add 10 units of regular insulin in 1L of fluid (D5LR or D5). Give IV infusion at 100 ml/hr with insulin 1 unit/hr.
    F. Postpartum Insulin Treatment: Monitor fasting and 2h postprandial glucose when tolerating PO intake or q4h while NPO. Start insulin if glucose exceeds 140–150 mg/dl. Normally only 50% of predelivery insulin dose is required.
XIV. Diabetic Ketoacidosis
    A. Symptoms of DKA include nausea, vomiting, abdominal pain, polyuria, polydipsia, hyperventilation, and obtundation.
    B. Laboratory Studies: Blood glucose ≥180. Positive serum ketone. pH <7.3, bicarbonate ≤15 mEq/L, base excess –4 or lower, anion gap ≥12.
    C. Late decelerations on fetal heart tracing normally will resolve after DKA is corrected.
    D. Treatment of Diabetic Ketoacidosis
        1. Glucose and electrolytes q2h
        2. Regular insulin loading dose 0.2–0.4 U/kg. Maintenance 2–10 U/hr
        3. Normal saline for a total replacement of 4–6L in first 12hr (1 L in first hr, 500–1,000 ml for 2–4h, then 250 ml/h until BP improved)
        4. 5% dextrose in NS when glucose is less than 250 mg/dl
        5. If potassium is normal or low, add KCL 40–60 mEq/L. If potassium level is high, wait until level drops to normal then add KCL
        6. Bicarbonate 1 amp (44 mEq) should be added to 1 L of 0.45 normal saline if pH is <7.10.

Respiratory Diseases

I. Influenza
A. Caused by influenza A or B during winter. Influenza causes 5–15% of URIs.
B. Pregnant women should receive inactivated vaccine. The influenza vaccine is safe in any trimester. Influenza vaccination begins in September. Immunity develops in two weeks.
C. **Diagnosis of Influenza**
   1. During influenza season, any patient with fever, cough or sore throat should be assumed to have influenza.
   2. Rapid influenza diagnostic tests of nasopharyngeal swab require less than 30 minutes, but have low sensitivity (40–60%).
   3. PCR test requires 1–6 hours to obtain results and is highly sensitive and specific.
   4. Viral cell cultures require 1–10 days.
D. **Treatment**
   1. During flu season, flu treatment should be started based on symptoms of fever, cough or sore throat. Influenza testing is not necessary.
   2. Neuraminidase inhibitors: oseltamivir (Tamiflu) 75 mg po qd for 5days; zanamivir (Relenza) 10 mg (2 inhalations) 2 times a day for 5 days.

II. Tuberculosis
A. **Targeted TB Testing**
   1. Conduct TB testing on high-risk groups.
   2. Tuberculosis screening consists of interferon gamma release assays (QuantiFERON). IFN-gamma is more specific and is preferred for pregnant women.
B. **Evaluation of Pregnant Women for TB**
   1. A negative QuantiFERON test requires no further evaluation, unless the patient has recently been exposed to tuberculosis.
   2. QuantiFERON test is positive in second or third trimester, perform chest X-ray with an abdominal shield. If the QuantiFERON test is positive in first trimester, delay chest X-ray until second trimester unless the patient has recent contact or is HIV positive.
   3. If chest X-ray normal with no recent contact or HIV positive, delay therapy for LTBI until 3–4 months postpartum.

III. Community-Acquired Pneumonia (CAP)
A. Community-acquired pneumonia occurs in 1 per 1,000 pregnancies.
B. **Pathogens**
   1. Bacterial causes of community-acquired pneumonia include Streptococcus pneumonia, which accounts for 50% of community acquired pneumonias. Other common bacteria include Haemophilus influenzae, Mycoplasma pneumoniae, Staphylococcus aureus, and Chlamydia pneumoniae. Unusual causes of community-acquired pneumonia include Pseudomonas aeruginosa, Legionella, Klebsiella, B. pertussis, and E. coli.
   2. Influenza A and B and varicella-zoster may cause pneumonia
C. **Clinical Evaluation**
   1. Symptoms of pneumonia include fever, chills, cough, sputum, dyspnea, chest pain, headache, fatigue, myalgia, and vomiting
   2. Physical signs of pneumonia include tachypnea, crackles, and a pleural rub
   3. Chest X-ray is diagnostic.

4. **Laboratory Studies:** CBC, metabolic panel, sputum Gram stain and culture, and blood culture

D. **Treatment**
1. Maintain PO_2 >70 mmHg.
2. Antibiotics should be continued for at least 5 days.
3. **Empiric IV Antibiotic Regimens**
   a) Ceftriaxone (Rocephin) 1g IV q24h and azithromycin (Zithromax) 500 mg IV q24h.
   b) Fluoroquinolones can be used in pregnancy. Fetal cartilage damage has not been reported in humans. Levofloxacin 750 mg IV q24h or moxifloxacin 400 mg IV q24h.

IV. Asthma

A. Asthma affects 8% of pregnancies. Severe asthma is associated with preeclampsia, preterm birth, and low birth weight.

B. **Mild Intermittent Asthma**
1. Brief (<1h) symptomatic exacerbations with ≤2 episodes/week with nocturnal symptoms ≤2 per month and PEFR or FEV_1 ≥80% of predicted when asymptomatic
2. Treatment of mild intermittent-asthma is a short-acting β_2-agonist, such as albuterol

C. **Mild Persistent Asthma**
1. >2 episodes per week but not daily with nocturnal symptoms >2/month, and PEFR or FEV_1 ≥80%
2. Management of mild persistent asthma is a low-dose inhaled steroid and a β_2-agonist inhaler as needed.

D. **Moderate Persistent Asthma**
1. Daily symptoms. Nocturnal symptoms >1 per week; PEFR or FEV_1 60 to 80% of predicted, and requires regular medications to control symptoms
2. Treatment of moderate persistent asthma is a medium-dose inhaled steroid and a long-acting β_2-agonist inhaler, such as salmeterol

E. **Severe Persistent Asthma**
1. Continuous symptoms with frequent exacerbations, which limit activity levels; PEFR or FEV_1 ≤ 60% of predicted, and regular oral corticosteroids are required to control symptoms
2. Treatment of severe persistent asthma is high-dose inhaled steroids, salmeterol, albuterol, and oral steroids.

F. **Treatment of Asthma Exacerbation**
1. Oxygen to maintain O_2 saturation >95%. Measure ABG if O_2 saturation is <90%.
2. Albuterol 2–4 puffs every 20 minutes up to 1 hour or terbutaline 0.25 mg SC every 15 min for 3 doses
3. SVN or BiPAP: 2.5 mg of albuterol in 3 ml normal saline q20 min. Ipratropium 500 mcg can be added for severe exacerbation.
4. Methylprednisolone (Solu-Medrol) 60–80 mg IQ every 6–8 hours, or IV hydrocortisone 2 mg/kg IV q4h, or prednisone 60–120 mg PO once a day
5. **Criteria for intubation and ICU admission:** PO_2 ≤60, PCO_2 ≥ 45, pH < 7.35, maternal exhaustion, and altered consciousness
6. For mild exacerbation, patient may be discharged if wheezing is completely resolved and fetal heart tracing is reassuring. Patient should be prescribed albuterol and inhaled steroids.

G. **Treatment of Asthma in Labor**
1. Continue albuterol by inhaler or nebulizer q2-4h as needed
2. Hydrocortisone 50–100 mg IV q8h until 24h after delivery to prevent adrenal crisis.

3. Pain management: epidural anesthesia is recommended for pain control. Fentanyl is preferred over morphine.

H. **Commonly Used Inhaled Corticosteroids**
   1. **Budesonide (Pulmicort)**
      a) Pulmicort Flexhaler: 90 mcg and 180 mcg per inhalation
      b) 1-4 puffs 2 times a day regimen. Budesonide is the preferred agent in pregnancy.
   2. **Beclomethasone (QVAR)**. Dose per puff: 40 mcg and 80 mcg.1-4 puffs bid.
   3. **Flunisolide (AeroBid)**. 80 mcg per inhalation. 1-4 puffs bid.
   4. **Fluticasone (Flovent)**. Flovent HFA: 44 mcg/inhalation (10.6 g); 110 mcg/inhalation (12 g); 220 mcg/inhalation (12 g). 1-4 puffs bid.

I. **Short Acting Inhaled β-Agonists - Albuterol Acute or Severe Exacerbation of Asthma**
   1. MDI: 4-8 puffs every 20 minutes for up to 4 hours, then every 1-4 hours as needed
   2. Solution for nebulization: 2.5-5 mg every 20 minutes for 3 doses, then 2.5-10 mg every 1-4 hours as needed, or 10-15 mg/hour by continuous nebulization.

J. **Combination Therapy with Inhaled Corticosteroids and Long-acting β-Agonist**
   1. **Fluticasone/salmeterol (Advair)**
      a) Advair Diskus: one inhalation twice daily, morning and evening, 12 hours apart. Maximum dose: fluticasone 500 mcg/salmeterol 50 mcg per inhalation (2 inhalations/day).
      b) Advair HFA: two inhalations twice daily, morning and evening, 12 hours apart. Maximum dose: fluticasone 230 mcg/salmeterol 21 mcg per inhalation (4 inhalations/day). Venous Thromboembolism

V. Venous Thromboembolism in Pregnancy
A. Pregnancy and the postpartum period are increased risk for venous thromboembolism, which includes pulmonary embolism and deep vein thrombosis.
B. Venous thromboembolism in pregnancy is 5 times more common than in nonpregnant women due to a hypercoagulable state, venous stasis, and vascular injury during delivery.
C. Pulmonary embolism accounts for 10.2% of maternal deaths.

II. Deep Vein Thrombosis
A. **Clinical Presentation:** DVT presents with sudden onset of pain and swelling in a lower extremity. The calf may be tender and warm to palpation. Homan sign is calf pain on stretching.
B. **Diagnosis**
   1. Venous compression ultrasound and color Doppler are the main imaging modalities for the diagnosis of deep vein thrombosis.
   2. D-dimer alone does not reliably predict venous thromboembolism. Negative D-dimer is useful in excluding venous thromboembolism.

III. Pulmonary Embolism
A. Pulmonary embolism may present with tachycardia, tachypnea, dyspnea, cough, chest pain, or hemoptysis.
B. **Imaging and Diagnosis**
   1. Spiral CT pulmonary angiography (CTPA) using is the gold standard for diagnosis of PE.
   2. Chest X-ray, ECG, D-dimer, and venous ultrasound of lower extremities may be abnormal.

IV. Treatment of Acute Venous Thromboembolism
A. If acute PE is suspected, immediately start unfractionated heparin or low molecular weight heparins.

B. Initial treatment is IV unfractionated heparin if delivery, surgery or thrombolysis may be necessary. Unfractionated heparin is given in a loading dose 70 units/kg IV (5,000 units), then 1,000 units/hr to aPTT of 1.5–2.5 times control (check aPTT q4–6h). Unfractionated heparin and low molecular weight heparins can be reversed with protamine.

C. If a deep vein thrombosis alone is suspected, may wait to initiate therapeutic anticoagulation after duplex confirmation of deep vein thrombosis.

D. Anticoagulation with adjusted-dose regimens is continued for at least 4 months.

E. **Pharmacological Regimens for Anticoagulation**

F. **Therapeutic-dose or Adjusted-dose Regimens**
   1. Enoxaparin (Lovenox) 1 mg/kg subcutaneous injection every 12 hours
   2. Dalteparin (Fragmin) 200 units/kg every 24 hours or 100 units/kg SC every 12 hours
   3. Tinzaparin (Innohep)175 units/kg SC q24h
   4. Unfractionated heparin ≥10,000 units SC q12h titrate to aPTT 1.5–2.5

G. **Prophylactic-dose or Low-dose Regimens**
   1. Enoxaparin 40 mg SC qd or 1 mg/kg/day
   2. Dalteparin 5,000 units SC qd or 2,500 units 2 times a day or 100 units/kg/day
   3. Tinzaparin 4,500 units SC qd.
   4. Unfractionated heparin 5,000–10,000 units q12h SC.
   5. Unfractionated heparin 5,000–7,500 units q12h SC during first trimester; 7,500–10,000 during second trimester; 10,000 during third trimester.

H. **Anticoagulant Monitoring**
   1. **Low molecular weight heparins:** Maintain antifactor Xa levels between 0.6 and 1.0 IU/ml 4h after an injection. Routine monitoring is not required.
   2. **Unfractionated Heparin:** Maintain the aPTT at 1.5–2.5 times control 4–6h after injection. Assess platelets weekly for 3 weeks for heparin-induced thrombocytopenia.

I. **Anticoagulation During Labor and Delivery**
   1. Withhold low molecular weight heparins for >24h for 10–12h before spinal or epidural anesthesia.
   2. Switch from low molecular weight heparins to unfractionated heparin in the last month of pregnancy.
   3. Low molecular weight heparins or unfractionated heparin can be discontinued 24 hours before induction of labor or scheduled cesarean.
   4. Protamine sulfate is used if rapid reversal of anticoagulation is needed.

V. **Postpartum Treatment**

A. Start low molecular weight heparins/unfractionated heparin 6–12h after cesarean and 4–6h after vaginal delivery.

B. If venous thromboembolism has developed in current pregnancy, the patient needs 3–6 months of anticoagulation postpartum. Start warfarin 5–10 mg PO qd after delivery and assess INR daily. Low molecular weight heparins/unfractionated heparin and warfarin are given together for the first 3–7 days until INR reaches 2.0–3.0 for 2 days. Then assess INR 2–3 times a week for 2 weeks.

C. Breastfeeding is safe while on warfarin or heparin. Progestins and the intrauterine system are safe while on warfarin or heparin. Estrogen containing pills are contraindicated while on warfarin or heparin.

VI. Antiphospholipid Syndrome
   A. Antiphospholipid antibodies are seen in 5% of healthy, pregnant women. Anticardiolipin antibodies (aCLs) are more prevalent than lupus anticoagulant. Lupus anticoagulant is associated with a greater risk of venous thromboembolism.
   B. Antiphospholipid antibodies are frequently found in patients with lupus and other autoimmune disorders. Systemic lupus erythematosus with positive antiphospholipid antibodies is high risk for venous thromboembolism.
   C. **Diagnosis of Antiphospholipid Syndrome**
      1. Pregnancy morbidity: ≥1 unexplained deaths of a normal fetus at ≥10 weeks; ≥1 premature birth before 34 weeks due to severe preeclampsia or uteroplacental insufficiency.
      2. Or ≥3 unexplained consecutive spontaneous abortions before 10 weeks.
   D. **Laboratory Criteria**
      1. Lupus anticoagulant present on ≥2 occasions 12 weeks apart.
      2. Anticardiolipin antibodies present in medium or high titers on ≥2 occasions 12 weeks apart.
      3. Anti-β2-glycoprotein-1 antibody present in titer above the 99th percentile on ≥2 occasions 12 weeks apart.
   E. **Indications for Screening for Antiphospholipid Syndrome**
      1. History of fetal loss or SAB (<10 weeks)
      2. History of unexplained venous thromboembolism, a new venous thromboembolism during pregnancy, or history of venous thromboembolism
   F. **Treatment**
      1. Antiphospholipid syndrome and a history of stillbirth or recurrent fetal loss but no prior thrombotic history is treated with prophylactic doses of heparin and low-dose aspirin during pregnancy and 6 weeks of postpartum.
      2. Antiphospholipid syndrome and a thrombotic event is treated with prophylactic heparin throughout pregnancy and 6 weeks postpartum.
      3. Antiphospholipid syndrome without a thrombotic event is treated with clinical surveillance or prophylactic heparin antepartum in addition to 6 weeks of postpartum anticoagulation.
VII. Thrombophilias are associated with venous thromboembolism.
   A. **Indication for Thrombophilia Screening**
      1. A personal history of venous thromboembolism
      2. A first-degree relative with a history of high-risk thrombophilia or venous thromboembolism before age 50 years.
   B. **Inherited Thrombophilias**
      1. Inherited thrombophilias include factor V Leiden (FVL), prothrombin G20210A mutation, antithrombin III deficiency, protein C deficiency, and protein S deficiency.
      2. FVL mutation is the most frequent type of inherited thrombophilia, occurring in 5% of Europeans. The FVL mutation results in activated protein C resistance.
      3. Thrombophilia screening panel should be done 6 weeks after the thrombotic event while not pregnant and not taking anticoagulant or hormone.
      4. Protein S level of less than 30% in second trimester and less than 24% in the third trimester may be consistent with protein S deficiency.
   C. **Acquired Thrombophilias** include lupus anticoagulant and anticardiolipin antibodies

D. **Treatment of Low-risk thrombophilia without previous venous thromboembolism**
   1. Antenatal managements surveillance without anticoagulation or prophylactic low molecular weight heparin or unfractionated heparin
   2. Postpartum: surveillance without anticoagulation therapy or postpartum anticoagulation therapy if patient has additional risk factors

E. **Low-risk thrombophilia with a single previous episode of venous thromboembolism—Not receiving long-term anticoagulation therapy**
   1. Antenatal management with prophylactic or intermediate-dose low molecular weight heparin/unfractionated heparin or surveillance without anticoagulation therapy
   2. Postpartum management with anticoagulation therapy or intermediate-dose low molecular weight heparin/unfractionated heparin

F. **High-risk thrombophilia without previous venous thromboembolism**
   1. Antenatal management with prophylactic low molecular weight heparin or unfractionated heparin
   2. Postpartum management with postpartum anticoagulation therapy

G. **High-risk thrombophilia with a single previous episode of venous thromboembolism—Not receiving long-term anticoagulation therapy**
   1. Antenatal management with prophylactic, intermediate-dose, or adjusted-dose low molecular weight heparin or unfractionated heparin regimen
   2. Postpartum anticoagulation therapy or adjusted-dose low molecular weight heparin or unfractionated heparin for 6 weeks

H. **No thrombophilia with previous single episode of venous thromboembolism associated with transient risk factor that is no longer present—Excludes pregnancy- or estrogen-related risk factor**
   1. Antenatal management with surveillance without anticoagulation
   2. Postpartum management with postpartum anticoagulation therapy

I. **No thrombophilia with prior episode of venous thromboembolism associated with transient risk factor that was pregnancy- or estrogen-related**
   1. Antenatal management is prophylactic-dose low molecular weight heparin or unfractionated heparin
   2. Postpartum management is postpartum anticoagulation therapy

J. **No thrombophilia with prior episode of venous thromboembolism without risk factor —Not receiving long-term anticoagulation therapy**
   1. Antenatal management is prophylactic-dose low molecular weight heparin or unfractionated heparin
   2. Postpartum management is postpartum anticoagulation therapy

K. **Thrombophilia or no thrombophilia with two or more episodes of venous thromboembolism—Not receiving long-term anticoagulation therapy**
   1. Antenatal management is prophylactic or therapeutic-dose low molecular weight heparin or unfractionated heparin
   2. Postpartum management is anticoagulation with therapeutic-dose low molecular weight heparin/unfractionated heparin for 6 weeks

L. **Thrombophilia or no thrombophilia with two or more venous thromboemboli—Receiving long-term anticoagulation therapy**
   1. Antenatal management is therapeutic-dose, low molecular weight heparin or unfractionated heparin.
   2. Postpartum management is long-term anticoagulation.

Heart Disease in Pregnancy

Women with cardiovascular conditions are at high risk for spontaneous abortion, preterm birth, and intrauterine growth restriction.

I. **Cardiovascular Changes in Pregnancy**
   A. Pregnancy causes a 40% increase in blood volume by 32 weeks' gestation. There is a 30% increase in cardiac output by 25–30 weeks. The heart rate increases by 17% in pregnancy.
   B. Vascular resistance declines during pregnancy until the second trimester.

II. **Cardiovascular Conditions**
   A. **Peripartum Cardiomyopathy**
      1. Incidence is 1 per 2,000–4,000 live births. Cardiomyopathy is much more frequent in Africans.
      2. Cardiomyopathy presents with dyspnea, fatigue, jugular venous distention during pregnancy and postpartum.
      3. **Diagnosis**
         a) Heart failure occurs in the last month of pregnancy or 5 months postpartum.
         b) Echocardiographic left ventricular dysfunction: ejection fraction <45%.
      4. **Treatment of Peripartum Hypertension**
         a) Furosemide, hydralazine, β-blockers, digoxin in pregnancy, ACE inhibitors postpartum, and anticoagulants.
         b) Future pregnancy is contraindicated if left ventricular function is abnormal.
   B. **Congenital Heart Diseases**
      1. Congenital heart disease is the most frequent heart condition in pregnancy.
      2. Congenital heart diseases are usually corrected in infancy. If untreated, large ventricular septal defect, atrial septal defect, and PDA can cause right-to-left shunt because of increased pulmonary resistance (Eisenmenger syndrome).
   C. **Valvular Heart Diseases**
      1. Valvular heart disease commonly results from rheumatic fever, congenital lesions, and degenerative changes.
      2. Women with prosthetic valves must use anticoagulation.
      3. **Valvular Heart Lesions Associated With High Maternal and/or Fetal Risk**
         a) Severe aortic stenosis with or without symptoms
         b) Aortic regurgitation with New York Heart Association class III–IV symptoms
         c) Mitral stenosis with NYHA class II–IV symptoms
         d) Mitral regurgitation with NYHA functional class III–IV symptoms
         e) Aortic and/or mitral valve disease resulting in severe pulmonary hypertension.
         f) Aortic and/or mitral valve disease with severe left ventricular dysfunction (ejection fraction <0.4).
         g) Mechanical prosthetic valve requiring anticoagulation
         h) Marfan syndrome with aortic regurgitation.
   D. **Coronary Artery Disease**
      1. Coronary artery disease is rare in pregnancy. Coronary artery disease is a major risk of pregnancy-related death.

2. Coronary artery disease presents with intense chest pain (burning, tightening or sharp), shortness of breath, sweating or palpitations. Pain may radiate to left arm, shoulder, neck or jaw.
3. Laboratory Evaluation: ECG and troponin I
4. Treatment: percutaneous coronary stent or CABG. Aspirin and clopidogrel are standard therapy. Statins and ACE inhibitors are contraindicated in pregnancy.
5. Delivery: Delivery should be delayed for 2–3 weeks after a myocardial infarction.

III. General Cardiac Care in Pregnancy

A. Antepartum Care
1. Order echocardiogram if cardiac disease is suspected.
2. Induce labor if the cervix is favorable and avoid prolonged labor.

B. Intrapartum Care
1. Monitor strict I&O in labor. Place patient in the left lateral position and supplement oxygen. Monitor pulse oximetry and arterial line.
2. Epidural anesthesia minimizes hemodynamic deterioration caused by pain.
3. Avoid maternal pushing by using low forceps or vacuum.

C. Postpartum Care
1. Infuse oxytocin. Avoid Methergine because Methergine may cause hypertension.
2. Careful diuresis postpartum.

D. Antibiotic Prophylaxis to Prevent Bacterial Endocarditis during Labor
1. Infective endocarditis prophylaxis is not recommended for vaginal or cesarean delivery except for cyanotic cardiac disease, or prosthetic valves. Antibiotic regimens for endocarditis prophylaxis are administered 30–60 minutes before delivery.
   a) Ampicillin 2g IV. Cefazolin or Ceftriaxone (Rocephin) 1g IV. If enterococcus needs to be covered, use penicillin, ampicillin, piperacillin or vancomycin
   b) If allergic to penicillin or ampicillin, use cefazolin or Ceftriaxone (Rocephin) for patients with history of rash allergy. Otherwise, use clindamycin 600 mg IV
   c) Oral regimen: amoxicillin 2g PO.

Thyroid Diseases

I. Thyroid Physiology in Pregnancy
A. Thyroid-binding globulin, total T3 and total T4 are increased in pregnancy because of hCG stimulation of TSH receptors
B. Free T3 and T4 are normal
C. Low TSH may occur in 15% of patients in the first trimester of normal pregnancy

II. Hyperthyroidism (Grave's Disease) . Fetal complications of hyperthyroidism include intrauterine growth restriction, preeclampsia, preterm labor, or pregnancy loss.

A. Diagnosis
1. Goiter, ophthalmopathy, and inability to gain weight
2. Thyroid storm and maternal cardiac failure are rare
3. Laboratory Studies: low TSH and elevated free T4

B. Medications
1. Thioamides: propylthiouracil (PTU) 100–150 mg PO q8h, max 600 mg/day or methimazole 10–20 mg PO 2 times a day

2. Both propylthiouracil and methimazole are associated with fetal goiter and hypothyroidism. The goal is to maintain free T4 in the upper 1/3 of normal

3. Propylthiouracil is preferred in early pregnancy because PTU is associated with fewer congenital malformations than methimazole

4. Propylthiouracil results in transient leukopenia in 10% of patients and agranulocytosis in 0.2%. Check a CBC if the patient has sore throat or fever.

5. Propranolol 20–40 mg PO q6h is used for symptomatic relief.

C. Surgery and Thyroid Ablation
1. Thyroidectomy is infrequently used in pregnancy and is indicated if the patient cannot tolerate thioamides.
2. Iodine-131 is contraindicated because I-131 destroys fetal thyroid tissue.

III. Subclinical Hyperthyroidism
A. Decreased TSH. Normal T4 and T3
B. No need to treat. Repeat labs in 6–12 weeks

IV. Hypothyroidism
A. Universal screening for hypothyroidism in pregnancy is not recommended.
B. Screening for hypothyroidism is indicated if patient has family history of thyroid disease, on thyroid medications, presence of goiter, history of neck radiation, postpartum thyroid dysfunction, infant with thyroid disease, or type 1 diabetes

C. Overt Hypothyroidism
1. Hypothyroidism is associated with pregnancy induced hypertension, preterm labor, low birth weight, placenta abruption, and stillbirth
2. Laboratory Studies: Low free T4 and elevated TSH
3. **Treatment**. Levothyroxine starting 50–100 µg qd, measure TSH every 4 weeks, increase levothyroxine in increments of 25 µg to achieve a normal TSH.

V. Subclinical Hypothyroidism
A. Asymptomatic patient with elevated TSH but normal free T4 and T3. Repeat labs in 6–12 weeks.

VI. Hyperthyroidism Related to Hyperemesis
A. Increased T3 and T4, low TSH
B. Hyperthyroidism resolves spontaneously with hyperemesis at 10–14 weeks. Treatment is symptomatic.

VII. Postpartum Thyroiditis
A. Hyperthyroidism (1–4 m) occurs first, followed by hypothyroidism (4–8 m).
B. Postpartum thyroiditis resolves 12 months postpartum.
C. Symptoms of hyperthyroidism are treated with propranolol. Symptoms hyperthyroidism are treated with levothyroxine.

Hepatic Diseases

I. Intrahepatic Cholestasis of Pregnancy
A. Risk factors for intrahepatic cholestasis of pregnancy include previous history of ICP, chronic hepatitis C, and multiple gestations.
B. Intrahepatic cholestasis of pregnancy causes intense pruritus in the third trimester. Serum bile acids, alkaline phosphatase, bilirubin and transaminases are elevated
C. Laboratory Studies: Fasting bile acids are >3 times normal. The AST/ALT, bilirubin, and a hepatitis panel should be checked.

D. Complications of ICP include preterm delivery, meconium staining of amniotic fluid, and fetal demise.

E. **Treatments for Pruritus**

   1. **Reduction of bile acids:** Ursodeoxycholic acid 300 mg po 2 times a day and increase to 600 mg 2 times a day if needed.

   2. **Antihistamines**
      a) Hydroxyzine (Vistaril, Atarax) 25–100 mg po four times a day prn
      b) Diphenhydramine (Benadryl) 25–50 mg po q4–6h

F. **Antenatal Surveillance and Early Delivery**

   1. ICP antepartum testing includes twice weekly nonstress test and amniotic fluid index measurements

   2. Patients with ICP should deliver at 37–38 weeks if fetal lung maturity positive.

II. Acute Fatty Liver of Pregnancy

A. Acute fatty liver of pregnancy is a rare condition, which causes nausea, fatigue, headache, or upper abdominal discomfort. Acute fatty liver of pregnancy may rapidly progress to jaundice, seizure, renal failure, and coagulopathy.

B. **Laboratory Studies:** Hypoglycemia, elevated liver enzymes, bilirubin, ammonia, and creatinine, prolonged INR.

C. Acute hepatitis A and B is associated with highly elevated AST and ALT (>1,000), and increased bilirubin (>5). Symptoms of acute hepatitis C are less severe than acute fatty liver, and elevations of liver enzymes are mild in hepatitis C. Liver biopsy demonstrates fatty infiltration and mitochondrial dysfunction.

D. Treatment is delivery and supportive care.

III. Hepatitis

A. **Hepatitis A**

   1. Hepatitis A is transmitted by fecal-oral transmission because of poor hygiene and sanitation. Hepatitis A vaccination may be administered in pregnancy for postexposure prophylaxis.

   2. Positive IgM antibody indicates acute hepatitis. Positive hepatitis A IgG indicates prior infection or vaccination.

   3. Hepatitis A is a self-limited disease, and no antiviral treatment is given.

B. **Hepatitis B** may be transmitted by blood and sexual contact. 10% become chronically infected with positive HBsAg. 15% of patients with chronic hepatitis B develop persistent hepatitis and cirrhosis.

C. **Treatment of HBsAg Positive Patients:** Serologic testing includes hepatitis B surface antibody (anti-HBs), total hepatitis B core antibody (anti-HBc), IgM antibody to hepatitis B core antigen (IgM anti-HBc), HBeAg, and hepatitis B viral DNA.

D. **Perinatal Transmission**

   1. 40% of infants born to women with hepatitis B become infected. Persistent infection occurs in 95% of infected infant.

   2. Newborns of carrier mothers should be given HBIG and hepatitis B virus vaccine to reduce perinatal transmission by 95%.

   3. Antiviral therapy reduces perinatal transmission: lamivudine 100 mg po qd beginning at 28 weeks to birth or 1 month after birth; HBIG 100–200 mg at 28, 32, and 36 gestational weeks.

   4. Cesarean does not prevent hepatitis B virus transmission. Avoid artificial rupture of membranes and fetal scalp electrodes in labor.

   5. Breastfeeding is not contraindicated in hepatitis B.

E. **Hepatitis C** is transmitted by blood products and IV drug use. 50% of patients with hepatitis C infection progress to chronic hepatitis. Diagnoses of hepatitis C is by antibody to HCV.

F. **Prenatal care:** Antiviral therapy is not advised during pregnancy.

G. **Perinatal Transmission**
   1. The rate of perinatal transmission is 2%, which is less than for hepatitis B.
   2. Labor and delivery: Cesarean section is indicated for obstetric indications only. Artificial rupture of membranes and fetal scalp electrodes should be avoided.
   3. Breastfeeding is safe with hepatitis C.

Rheumatic Diseases

I. **Rheumatoid Arthritis**
   A. Symptoms of rheumatoid arthritis improve in pregnancy because of pregnancy-related immunologic changes.
   B. Rheumatoid arthritis is not usually associated with adverse pregnancy outcomes.
II. **Systemic Lupus Erythematosus**
   A. SLE is associated with fetal loss and preterm birth.
   B. Risk factors for fetal loss include proteinuria >500 mg/24h. Antiphospholipid syndrome, thrombocytopenia (platelet <150,000), and a blood pressure >140/90.
   C. **Treatment of Systemic Lupus Erythematosus in Pregnancy**
      1. **Preconception Counseling**
         a) Pregnancy in SLE is relatively contraindicated if the creatinine is 1.5–2 mg/dl and absolutely contraindicated if the creatinine is >2 mg/dl.
         b) Complications of SLE in pregnancy include preeclampsia, spontaneous abortion, preterm birth, intrauterine growth restriction, and fetal demise.
      2. **Prenatal Care**
         a) Laboratory evaluation: ultrasound, CBC, metabolic panel, uric acid, C3 and C4, lupus anticoagulant antibody, anticardiolipin antibody, anti-SSA (Ro), anti-SSB (La), anti-DS DNA, 24-hr urine protein, and creatinine clearance
         b) Check fetal heart rate every 1–2 weeks if anti-SSA and/or anti-SSB positive and obtain fetal echocardiogram if bradycardia is detected.
         c) Perform ultrasound every 3–4 weeks to monitor fetal growth.
         d) Monitor weight gain and blood pressure. Repeat labs every 1–2 months.
         e) Antepartum testing should start at 28–34 weeks. Early delivery is appropriate.
      3. **Medications for Rheumatic Diseases**
         a) **NSAIDs** are safe in the second trimester. Avoid NSAIDs and high-dose aspirin after 32 weeks because of premature closure of ductus arteriosus.
         b) **Corticosteroids**
            (1) Prednisone is the safest steroid in pregnancy because only 10% passes the placenta, as compared to free passage of betamethasone and dexamethasone.
            (2) Steroids may cause cleft palate. Avoid steroids in the first trimester.
         c) **Steroids in Labor**
            (1) Continue same regimen if patient takes prednisone <20 mg/day.

(2) If patient takes ≥20 mg of prednisone a day for ≥3 weeks, give 50–100 mg hydrocortisone IV every 8 hours for 24 hours to prevent adrenal crisis. Continue usual dose.
  d) **Drugs that can be used in pregnancy**
    (1) Hydroxychloroquine, sulfasalazine, azathioprine, and 6-mercaptopurine (6-MP) are safe in pregnancy.
    (2) Cyclosporine and tacrolimus can be given at low lose. Avoid in breastfeeding.
  e) **Drugs that cannot be used in pregnancy**
    (1) Methotrexate and other anti-neoplastics may cause congenital malformations.
    (2) TNF inhibitors and interleukin antagonists are not advised during pregnancy and breastfeeding.

Anemia and Thrombocytopenia

Anemia in pregnancy is hemoglobin <11 g/dL and hematocrit less than 33% in first and third trimester. Anemia is a hemoglobin <10.5 g/dL and hematocrit <32% in second trimester.

Ferritin is the most sensitive and specific test for iron deficiency. A ferritin <15 confirms the diagnosis of iron deficiency. Ferritin declines mildly in pregnancy and increases with inflammation. Total iron-binding capacity (TIBC) and serum iron are nonspecific. TIBC rises in 15% of normal pregnancies

I. **Iron Deficiency Anemia**
  A. Anemia in pregnancy is usually because of iron deficiency. Mild to moderate iron deficiency can be diagnosed and managed presumptively. CBC, serum iron level, and ferritin are diagnostic.
  B. Prenatal vitamins contain 27 mg of elemental iron, which satisfies the recommended daily dietary allowance.
II. **Oral iron preparations.** Ferrous sulfate 325 mg once a day to 3 times a day; ferrous fumarate 325 mg once a day to 3 times a day; ferrous gluconate 300 mg once a day to 3 times a day; or polysaccharide iron complex (Niferex) 150 mg once a day.
III. **Hemoglobinopathies**
  A. **Sickle Cell Disease**
    1. 1 in 600 African Americans has sickle cell disease and 1 in 12 carries the trait.
    2. Sickle cell disease is associated with preterm labor, premature rupture of membranes, intrauterine growth restriction, fetal demise, infections, and sickle cell crisis.
    3. Antepartum care: folic acid 4 mg/day. Maintain adequate fluid intake and avoid heavy exercise. Antenatal testing should begin at 32 weeks. Serial ultrasound for fetal growth
    4. Treatment of painful crisis: O_2, hydration, analgesia, and transfusion of packed red blood cells to maintain hemoglobin of 10 g/dl.
  B. **Thalassemia**
    1. β-thalassemia occurs in patients of Mediterranean or Middle Eastern descent. α-Thalassemia occurs in Southeast Asians.
    2. Hemoglobin electrophoresis is diagnostic for β-thalassemia, Hb S, Hb SS, Hb SC, and Hb AC. α-Thalassemia requires DNA-based testing.
    3. Pregnancy outcome is usually normal in thalassemia trait or minor. Iron replacement is contraindicated due to iron overload in thalassemia. Folate 1 mg once a day should be prescribed.

C. **Thrombocytopenia**
   1. **Gestational Thrombocytopenia**
      a) Platelets 50,000–120,000/mm^3
      b) Most common cause of low platelets in pregnancy
      c) Benign condition and no need for treatment
   2. **Immune Thrombocytopenic Purpura (ITP)**
      a) ITP is a platelet count less than 50,000/mm^3. Bleeding may occur if platelet count is less than 20,000/mm^3.
      b) Start treatment if platelets are less than 50,000/mm^3, and maintain platelet count at 100,000/mm^3
      c) Treatment of ITP is prednisone, 1 mg/kg/day po. Acute bleeding is managed with IV methylprednisolone 1–1.5 mg/kg
      d) Intravenous immunoglobulin: 400 mg/kg/d for 3 days or 1 g/kg/d for 2 days
      e) Platelet transfusion is reserved for life-threatening bleeding. Transfused platelets are rapidly destroyed.
      f) Splenectomy may be indicated if other therapies are unsuccessful.
      g) For Rh positive patient who failed other measures, give IV RhoGAM 50–75 µg.
   3. **Alloimmune Thrombocytopenia**
      a) Gestational-thrombocytopenia is the most common cause of severe fetal and neonatal thrombocytopenia. GT is because of maternal antibody against fetal platelets.
      b) Maternal platelets are normal.
      c) IVIG may be combined with prednisone to prevent fetal thrombocytopenia in future pregnancies.

Neurological Disorders

I. **Epilepsy**
   A. Pregnant epileptic patients may have seizures. Seizures are usually because of noncompliance with medication and low drug levels.
   B. Epilepsy increases the risk of intrauterine growth restriction, fetal demise, fetal anomalies, and preeclampsia.
   C. Valproic acid, phenytoin, phenobarbital, and carbamazepine are associated with fetal neural tube defects, heart defects, craniofacial defects, and developmental delay.
   D. **Treatment of Epilepsy in Pregnancy**
      1. Folic acid 4 mg daily should be prescribed for patients with a seizure disorder.
      2. Consider stopping antiepileptic drugs if patient has not had seizure for 2 years.
      3. Measure serum drug levels monthly. Drug levels will decrease as pregnancy progresses.
      4. Valproic acid, phenytoin, and phenobarbital should be avoided.
      5. Establish gestation age with early ultrasound and screen for neural tube defects with alpha fetoprotein and ultrasound at 16 weeks. Screen for cardiac defects at 18–22 weeks with target ultrasound and/or fetal echocardiogram and perform serial ultrasounds for fetal growth.
      6. Routine nonstress test and amniotic fluid index testing are not necessary
      7. Vitamin K is administered to prevent neonatal bleeding at 36 weeks; 10 to 20 mg po every day.

E. **Treatment of Status Epilepticus**
   1. Lorazepam (Ativan) 0.02 to 0.03 mg/kg IV, repeat as needed, maximum 0.1 mg/kg
   2. Fosphenytoin is a prodrug of phenytoin. Fosphenytoin is given as mg of phenytoin equivalent (PE). Loading dose 15–20 mg PE/kg at a rate of 100–150 mg PE/minute.
F. **First Generation Antiepileptic Drugs.** The frequency of embryopathy in first trimester with phenytoin is 21%, phenobarbital 27%, carbamazepine 14%, and polytherapy 28%.
G. **Phenytoin**
   1. Oral load: 400 mg, then 300 mg and 400 mg in 2 and 4 hr. Maintenance dose: 100 mg 3 times a day or extended-release 300 mg once a day.
   2. Fetal hydantoin syndrome is hypoplasia and ossification of the distal phalanges and craniofacial defect. Phenytoin causes maternal gingival hyperplasia, hirsutism, and CNS, liver, and bone marrow toxicity.
H. **Carbamazepine**
   1. 200 mg PO 2 times a day. Increase weekly by 200 mg/day to max 1,600 mg/day, divided 3 times a day or QID. Extended-release formulation is given 2 times a day.
   2. Carbamazepine is associated with fetal craniofacial and neural-tube defects. Maternal side-effects include dizziness, ataxia, blurred vision, hematologic toxicity, and hypersensitivity
I. **Valproic acid**
   1. Valproic acid should be avoided in pregnancy, especially during the first trimester.
   2. Neural tube defects occur in 1 in 20 pregnancies if exposed to valproic acid during the first 12 weeks.
J. **New Antiepileptic Drugs**
   1. Lamotrigine (Lamictal) may cause oral clefts. Dosing for immediate release formulations is 25 mg/day for weeks 1 and 2, then increase to 50 mg/day for weeks 3 and 4. Then every 1–2 weeks by 50 mg/day. Usual maintenance: 225–375 mg/day in 2 divided doses.
   2. Gabapentin (Neurontin): Start 300 mg qhs, increase to 300–600 mg 3 times a day, max 2,400 mg in long-term therapy
   3. Topiramate (Topamax): Associated with oral cleft; 25 mg 2 times a day week 1, 50 mg 2 times a day week 2, 75 mg 2 times a day week 3, 100 mg 2 times a day week 4, 150 mg 2 times a day week 5, then 200 mg 2 times a day as tolerated

II. **Migraine**
A. **Treatment of Acute Migraine**
   1. Acetaminophen (Tylenol) 1,000 mg PO or PR q4h
   2. Acetaminophen + aspirin + caffeine (Excedrin Migraine) 2 tabs q4–6h
   3. Opioids and antiemetic therapy
B. **Triptans**
   1. Indicated for moderate to severe migraine
   2. NSAIDs should be limited to 48 hours in the third trimester.

Skin Disorders

I. **Physiological Skin Changes**
A. **Hyperpigmentation**
   1. Hyperpigmentation causes linea nigra, darkening of the nipple and areola, and facial chloasma (melasma) because of elevated melanocyte-stimulating hormone or estrogen and progesterone.

2. Hyperpigmentation fades after pregnancy. The patient should avoid sun exposure. Topical hydroquinone or retinoid acid may be effective for persistent melasma after pregnancy.

B. Striae
1. Striae appear after the second trimester.
2. Striae usually fade over time but do not disappear completely.

C. Vascular Changes
1. Varicosities of lower extremities and vulva are common.
2. Telangiectasias, spider angioma, palmar erythema, and pyogenic granuloma are infrequent.

II. Dermatoses in Pregnancy

A. Pruritic Urticarial Papules and Plaques of Pregnancy (PUPPP)
1. PUPPP is the most common gestational dermatosis. PUPP occurs in primigravidas in the third trimester.
2. Lesions involve mid- and lower abdomen, buttocks, and proximal thighs. Red, pruritic, and urticarial papules from plaques.

B. Antipruritic Medications
1. Hydroxyzine 25–100 mg PO once a day to QID or prn. Diphenhydramine 25–50 mg PO q4–6h.
2. Topical triamcinolone or fluocinonide

C. Pruritus occurs in up to 14% of pregnancies. Treatment is oral antihistamines.

D. Pemphigoid Gestationis
1. Pemphigoid gestationis presents with urticarial papules around umbilicus and extremities. Lesions may form bullae.
2. 10% of fetus can be affected by PG because of maternal IgG crossing the placenta. Antepartum fetal assessment is indicated because growth restriction may occur.
3. ELISA is highly sensitive and specific for pemphigoid gestationis.
4. Topical corticosteroids are used for localized disease. Prednisone 20 mg po qd may be administered.

E. Pruritic Folliculitis of Pregnancy
1. Pemphigoid gestationis presents with papules and pustules around hair follicles in the third trimester.
2. Benzoyl peroxide and topical steroids are effective.

Urinary Tract Disorders

I. Asymptomatic Bacteriuria and Acute Cystitis
A. E. coli causes 70% of urinary tract infections. Other organisms include Klebsiella pneumoniae, Proteus, enterococci, Staphylococci, and group B streptococcus.
B. Urine cultures should be obtained pregnant women with UTI. Urine dipstick tests are insufficient for diagnosis of UTI in pregnancy.

C. Asymptomatic Bacteriuria
1. Asymptomatic bacteriuria is defined as isolation of a single organism of $\geq 10^5$ colonies/ml from a midstream clean-catch urine specimen, or $\geq 10^2$ colonies/ml from a catheterized specimen.
2. Asymptomatic bacteriuria in pregnancy requires treatment due to the risk of progression to pyelonephritis and the risk of preterm labor.

D. Acute Cystitis
1. Acute cystitis presents with dysuria, frequency, urgency, suprapubic pain, and hematuria.
2. Urine dipstick positive leukocyte esterase is 75% sensitive nitrite is 82% sensitivity. Urinalysis detects pyuria.

3. Urine culture: 10^2 colonies/ml on a midstream urine specimen in symptomatic women is diagnostic.

E. **Treatment**
1. Nitrofurantoin (Macrodantin) 100 mg q6h or nitrofurantoin dual-release (Macrobid) 100 mg q12h for 7 days. Nitrofurantoin is bacteriostatic. Avoid nitrofurantoin after 38 weeks, because of neonatal anemia. Single-dose treatment is not recommended during pregnancy.
2. Trimethoprim-sulfamethoxazole DS (Bactrim-DS, Septra DS) 160/800 mg 2 times a day for 3 days. Interferes with bilirubin binding in near-term neonates.
3. Cephalexin (Keflex) 250–500 mg q6h for 3d or amoxicillin 500 or 875 mg 2 times a day for 3 days. Less effective because of antibiotic resistance.
4. Fluoroquinolone, levofloxacin 250 mg qd for 3 days, gatifloxacin 200 mg qd, ciprofloxacin 250 mg 2 times a day, or norfloxacin 400 mg 2 times a day. Used for urinary tract infection resistant to other drugs.
5. Cefpodoxime 100 mg po for 3 days. Amoxicillin-clavulanate 500 mg 2 times a day for 3 days. Fosfomycin 3 grams po.

F. **Suppressive Regimens**
1. Suppressive therapy is indicated ≥2 cystitis episodes in a pregnancy.
2. Nitrofurantoin 100 mg qd is taken for the remainder of the pregnancy.

II. Pyelonephritis
A. 80% of pyelonephritis occurs on the right side
B. Dysuria, urgency, frequency, flank pain, fever, chills, and CVA tenderness, and septic shock
C. Uterine contractions or preterm labor
D. **Inpatient Treatment**
1. Assess CBC, BMP, and urine culture. Monitor fetal heart rate and uterine contractions. Hydration with IV fluids.
2. Ceftriaxone (Rocephin) 1–2 g IV q24h
3. If patient is septic or febrile 48 hours after initiation of antibiotics, add gentamycin 1.5 mg/kg q8h.
4. Admit tor ICU if signs of septic shock.
5. Renal ultrasound may be indicated to exclude obstruction or renal abscess. Modify the antibiotic regimen based on urine culture and susceptibility if no improvement by 48–72 hours.
6. Change to oral antibiotics for 14 days after afebrile for 24–48h.

E. **Outpatient Treatment**
1. Outpatient treatment is appropriate for mild symptoms, T ≤ 39.8, HR <100, no sepsis or preterm labor, and no underlying disease.
2. Ceftriaxone (Rocephin) 1g IM and second injection the next day. If responding, start cephalexin (Keflex) 500 mg q6h for 10 days.

F. **Suppressive Regimen**
1. Nitrofurantoin 100 mg PO qd for the remainder of pregnancy
2. Recheck urine culture monthly

III. Urolithiasis
A. **Presentation and Diagnosis**
1. A stone in the ureter presents with acute onset of flank or abdominal pain, and microscopic or gross hematuria. Obstruction may cause pyelonephritis.
2. Urinalysis, urine culture, and CBC with differential
3. Renal ultrasound may demonstrate a dilated ureter with distal obstruction. Ultrasound cannot detect stone less than 4 mm.

B. **Treatment**
1. Nephrolithiasis usually passes spontaneously.

2. Treatment is pain control with morphine and hydration. Antibiotics are given to prevent infection. Patients should strain their urine for several days. Stones are sent for analysis.
3. Lithotripsy is only used for nonpregnant patients and is not recommended in pregnancy.
4. If the stone does not pass, ureteroscopy and ureteral stenting are indicated.

HIV Infection in Pregnancy

I. Antepartum Care
A. HIV Screening
1. Universal HIV testing is completed at the first prenatal visit. For high-risk women, second test should be done during the third trimester.
2. If a patient presents in labor without third trimester test. She should be screened with a rapid HIV test.

B. Antepartum Care for HIV-infected Patients
1. Laboratory Studies: CD4, HIV RNA load, CBC, and metabolic panel. Assess HIV RNA level 2–4 weeks after starting therapy. Repeat CD4 and HIV RNA every 3 months. At 34–36 weeks, assess HIV RNA level to determine the mode of delivery.
2. Avoid amniocentesis. If amniocentesis is indicated, amniocentesis should be performed after initiation of antiretroviral therapy when HIV RNA levels are undetectable.

C. Principles of Antiretroviral Therapy
1. Antiretroviral therapy is advised to all pregnant patients to prevent perinatal HIV transmission.
2. Antiretroviral regimens should include NRTIs with high placental passage, such as zidovudine, lamivudine, emtricitabine, tenofovir, or abacavir.
3. Drug resistance testing should be performed before starting treatment.
4. Stavudine/didanosine may cause lactic acidosis and maternal/neonatal mortality. Nevirapine can cause severe liver toxicity.

D. Intrapartum Zidovudine
1. Intrapartum IV zidovudine should be given to HIV-infected women with HIV RNA ≥400 copies/ml near delivery, regardless of antepartum treatment or mode of delivery.
2. IV zidovudine is not required if the woman is receiving antiretroviral therapy with HIV RNA <400 copies/ml.
3. Zidovudine 2 mg/kg IV loading zone over 1 hour, then 1 mg/kg/hr until delivery.
4. For a scheduled cesarean, start IV zidovudine 3 hours before surgery.
5. Continue antiretrovirals during the intrapartum period.

II. HIV Transmission and Mode of Delivery
A. Scheduled cesarean delivery at 38 weeks is advised for women with HIV RNA >1,000 copies/ml to minimize perinatal transmission of HIV
B. Cesarean is not recommended if the woman is receiving antiretroviral therapy and the HIV RNA is <1,000 copies/ml.

III. Management of Labor
A. Avoid artificial rupture of membranes, fetal scalp electrodes, forceps, and vacuum delivery
B. Avoid Methergine in women receiving a protease inhibitors or nevirapine, efavirenz, etravirine.
C. Breastfeeding is contraindicated in HIV-infected mothers

Perinatal Infections

I. Toxoplasmosis
A. Toxoplasma gondii is an intracellular parasite, transmitted by under-cooked, contaminated meat or cat feces
B. Toxoplasmosis may be asymptomatic or may cause fever, malaise, myalgias, and lymphadenopathy

II. Diagnosis
A. Diagnosis of toxoplasmosis is by maternal serology for IgM and IgG
B. Fetal infection is diagnosed by amniotic PCR and fetal blood serology
C. Fetal ultrasound may demonstrate ventriculomegaly, microcephaly, in-tracranial calcification, hepatosplenomegaly, ascites, and intrauterine growth restriction

III. Treatment
A. Spiramycin reduces transmission of toxoplasmosis by 60%. Fetal infec-tion is treated with a multidrug regimen.

IV. Rubella
A. Vaccination against MMR is given to all children. All pregnant women are tested for rubella immunity.
B. Congenital rubella syndrome causes cataracts, deafness, heart defects, mental retardation, development delay, jaundice, and "blueberry muffin" skin lesions.
C. Maternal symptoms include mild fever, maculopapular rash, lymphade-nopathy, arthralgia, and abortion. Rubella may cause fetal malfor-mations in early pregnancy
D. Suspected infection is assessed with serial serology testing for IgG and IgM.

V. Cytomegalovirus
A. CMV is transmitted by blood, saliva, urine, and sex. CMV infection is usually asymptomatic or causes flu-like symptoms.
B. CMV is the most common congenital infection (0.2%). The transmission rate is 30% with possible severe sequelae with primary cytomegalovirus in first trimester. Third trimester infection is less severe. Fetal manifes-tations of CMV infection include intracranial calcifications, microcephaly, retardation, and chorioretinitis
C. Diagnosis is made by seroconversion or a 4-fold increase in IgG. Amni-otic fluid culture and PCR are used for fetal diagnosis.
D. Fetal ultrasound demonstrates calcifications in the liver and ventricles with increased size and echogenic bowel, ascites, and hydrops

VI. Genital Herpes
A. Herpes simplex virus is transmitted by direct and intimate contact. Pro-dromal symptoms of herpes include vulvar burning, pain, followed by painful vesicles. The neonatal infection rate is 60% if the fetus is deliv-ered through primary genital lesions. The risk of neonatal infection is 3% if the fetus is delivered through recurrent herpes.
B. **Prophylaxis**: for women with active recurrent genital herpes is acyclovir (Zovirax), 400 mg PO 3 times a day; or valacyclovir (Valtrex) 500 mg PO 2 times a day at 36-week gestation until delivery.
C. Cesarean delivery is indicated if lesions are present on the genitalia at time of delivery.

VII. Varicella Zoster
A. Varicella is transmitted by respiratory droplets and physical contact. Varicella is diagnosed by maculopapular pruritic rashes and vesicles and positive HVZ IgG and IgM.

B. Varicella increases maternal morbidity and mortality in pregnancy. Severe neonatal infection may develop if the mother is infected within 3 weeks of delivery.

C. Congenital varicella syndrome consists of skin scaring, limb hypoplasia, chorioretinitis, and microcephaly. Congenital varicella occurs in 2% of newborns if maternal infection occurred at 13–20 weeks.

D. Fetal ultrasound demonstrates intrauterine growth restriction, hydrops, echogenic foci in the liver and bowel, heart and limb defects, and microcephaly

E. Acyclovir is administered within 24h of the rash. Acyclovir does not prevent fetal disease.

F. Varicella-zoster immune globulin (VZIG) may be given within 96 hours of exposure.

VIII. **Parvovirus B19**

A. Parvovirus B19 is transmitted by respiratory or hand-to-mouth routes, resulting in a childhood exanthema known as erythema infectiosum. The exanthema is a reticular rash with a "slapped cheek" appearance. Parvovirus B19 may cause aplastic crisis

B. Severe fetal sequelae of parvovirus B19 infection include fetal loss, severe anemia, nonimmune hydrops, and stillbirth.

C. Maternal IgM and IgG serology is diagnostic

D. Fetal diagnosis of parvovirus B19 is by viral culture and PCR of amniotic fluid or tissue

E. The fetus is monitored with ultrasound. Intrauterine transfusion are used to treat hydrops and fetal aplastic crises.

IX. **Cytomegalovirus, Toxoplasmosis, Varicella, or Parvovirus B19 Exposure**

A. Positive serology for IgG indicates that the patient has had prior exposure and developed immunity. A positive IgM indicates newly acquired infection or recurrent infection.

B. After infection, ultrasound is indicated to assess fetal anatomy and establish dates.

Acute Abdomen in Pregnancy

I. **Appendicitis**

A. Appendicitis is the most common cause of acute abdomen in pregnancy. Appendicitis is less frequent during pregnancy than in the nonpregnant state.

B. **Diagnosis**

1. Appendicitis presents with acute onset of right lower abdominal pain and RLQ tenderness with nausea, vomiting, low-grade fever, rebound tenderness in RLQ, and leukocytosis

2. The differential diagnosis includes urinary tract infection, cholecystitis, renal and ureteral stones, adnexal torsion, preterm labor, and placenta abruption.

3. Ultrasound is the imaging modality in pregnancy less than 35 weeks.

C. **Treatment**

1. Surgery is indicated if appendicitis is suspected.

2. Ampicillin 2 gm IV q6h or 50 mg/kg q6h and Metronidazole (Flagyl) 500 mg IV q6h and gentamicin 2.5 mg/kg IV q8h.

3. Fetal monitoring is continued after surgery.

II. Gallbladder Disease
A. Biliary Colic
1. Biliary colic causes acute onset upper epigastric cramping, nausea, and vomiting. The patient is usually afebrile.
2. Tenderness is usually present in the right, upper quadrant.
3. The pain is constant and resolves in several hours. Biliary colic is caused by gallbladder stones or sludge, and biliary colic may progress to cholecystitis if cystic duct blockage is not relieved.

B. Acute Cholecystitis
1. Acute cholecystitis is the second most frequent surgical acute abdomen in pregnancy.
2. Symptoms of acute cholecystitis include severe RUQ or epigastric pain, which radiates to the right shoulder or back with anorexia, nausea, and vomiting.
3. Physical exam causes an ill appearance with fever, severe RUQ tenderness and guarding, and Murphy's sign.
4. Laboratory Studies: leukocytosis with increased bands and mildly elevated LFTs.
5. Ultrasound demonstrates gallstones establishes diagnosis of cholecystitis.
6. **Differential diagnosis:** severe preeclampsia, pancreatitis, appendicitis, pyelonephritis, peptic ulcer, or myocardial infarction.

C. Treatment
1. NPO, IV hydration and analgesia.
2. Ampicillin-sulbactam (Unasyn) 3 gm IV q6h PLUS Ceftriaxone (Rocephin) 1 gm IV q24h OR Cefotaxime (Claforan) 2 gm IV q8h
3. Recurrence is over 50% in the same pregnancy.
4. **Surgery.** Laparoscopic cholecystectomy in pregnancy is associated with better maternal and fetal outcomes.

III. Pancreatitis
A. Pancreatitis presents with upper epigastric pain with elevation of amylase and lipase.
B. Pancreatitis is usually caused by gallstones and choledocholithiasis. Alcoholism may also cause pancreatitis.
C. Treatment of pancreatitis by GI rest, IV hydration, and pain relief.

Pregnancy Termination

I. Surgical Abortion
A. **First trimester abortion with dilation and curettage** is most common method of terminating pregnancy <14 weeks gestation.
B. **Pre-operative evaluation:** Pregnancy test, pelvic exam, ultrasound for dating, and Rh factor testing
C. **Procedure:**
1. Anesthesia for dilator and curettage is conscious sedation with midazolam 2–3 mg and fentanyl. A paracervical block is placed with 1% lidocaine. Atropine prevents vasovagal syncope.
2. Cervical dilation is not needed if less than 7 weeks. If ≥7 weeks, cervical dilation is performed with metal dilators or vaginal misoprostol. Misoprostol 400 µg can be given vaginally or sublingually 2–3 hours before the procedure to dilate the cervix.
3. The size of the suction cannula is equal to the gestational age. The suction pressure should be 50–70 mm Hg
4. The issue should be floated in water to identify the villi. Give RhoGAM if Rh negative.

5. Infection prophylaxis is doxycycline 100 mg 1 hr before the procedure and 200 mg PO after the procedure.

D. **Second Trimester Abortion**

1. **Dilation and Evacuation**

   a) Dilation and evacuation is used for pregnancy termination after 14 weeks

   b) D&E is safer than intrauterine instillation up to 16 weeks.

   c) Multistage cervical dilation is needed with laminaria or Dilapan in advanced gestation. Special forceps, e.g., Sopher forceps, are required to destruct and retrieve fetal tissues under ultrasound guidance.

2. **Intact dilation and extraction** is also called "partial-birth abortion." Dilation and extraction involves decompression of the fetal calvarium after breech delivery of fetal body.

3. **Complications**

   a) Uterine perforation is managed by observation. A laparoscopy or laparotomy is performed if bowel injury or major intra-abdominal hemorrhage develops.

   b) Hemorrhage, retained product of conception, infection, and failure to recognize ectopic pregnancy are also possible complications.

4. **Medical Abortion**

   a) Mifepristone is used for up to 49 days of gestation, with a success rate 96%.

   b) Mifepristone is usually followed by misoprostol.

5. **Disadvantages**. Medical abortion is associated with prolonged pain, bleeding, nausea, vomiting, diarrhea, or low fever. Dilation and curettage is necessary if medical abortion is not successful.

6. **Protocols**

   a) Mifepristone 200 mg po

   b) Misoprostol can be given vaginally, orally, sublingually, or buccally 800 µg per vagina is effective.

      c) Misoprostol is given at same time with mifepristone.

GYNECOLOGY

General Gynecology

Contraception

I. Preprescription Counseling
A. Medical history to exclude any contraindication to estrogen use.
B. Assess blood pressure and BMI. Breast exam, Pap smear, sexually transmitted disease screening, and pelvic exam are not required.
C. Assess blood pressure and BMI. Breast exam, Pap smear, sexually transmitted disease screening, and pelvic exam are not required.
D. 7 to 13 packs of pills should be provided to improve continuation rates.

II. Relative Contraindications to Oral Contraceptives
A. History of hypertension, venous thromboembolic events, estrogen-dependent tumors, migraine with aura, and age 35 years and older who smoke or have a history of migraine.
B. Small risk for stroke and MI.

III. Noncontraceptive Benefits of Oral Contraceptives
A. 50% decrease in endometrial cancer; 40% reduction in ovarian cancer.
B. Regular menses with reduced flow. Reduction in dysmenorrhea and anemia.
C. Decreased ectopic pregnancy and decreased pelvic inflammatory disease.
D. Improved bone density, less endometriosis, less benign breast disease, ovarian cysts, acne, and hirsutism

IV. Starting an Oral Contraceptive
A. Quick start on the day of the clinic visit after negative pregnancy test. Use backup condom contraception for 1 week.
B. Start on the first Sunday after next menses begins. Use backup for 1 week
C. Start oral contraceptive on the first day of next menses

V. Which Pill to Choose
A. Combined oral contraceptives contain various dosages of ethinyl estradiol and different progestins (norethindrone, norethindrone acetate, levonorgestrel, norgestimate, and desogestrel). Desogestrel is a third generation progestin with the least androgenic activity. Desogestrel is associated with a higher rate of thromboembolism.
B. Very low dose pills, with <25 µg of estradiol, cause spotting or breakthrough bleeding. Very low dose pills are a good choice for perimenopausal women.
C. Yasmin and Yaz contain 3 mg of drospirenone (anti-mineralocorticoid) and are associated with a small amount of weight loss, BP reduction, hyperkalemia, and a 2- to 3-times higher risk of venous thromboembolism
D. Biphasic and triphasic pills mimic normal hormonal changes, but have no clinical differences compared to monophasics.
E. Extended regimens eliminate scheduled monthly bleeding and improve menstrual symptoms, but spotting may occur.
F. Progestin-only pill (mini-pill) prevents pregnancy by thickening cervical mucus and thinning the uterine lining. Ovulation is not consistently suppressed. Monthly menses and irregular spotting may occur. Pills should be taken at the same time every day.

VI. Missed Pills
A. If one pill is missed, take the missed pill as soon as possible and resume the normal schedule.
B. If two pills were missed in the first 2 weeks: take 2 pills a day for 2 days,

and then finish the pack.
C. If two pills were missed in the third week or 3 pills were missed at any other times: start a new pack and use a back-up method of contraception.

VII. Breakthrough Bleeding
A. Breakthrough bleeding occurs in 10% of patients in the first 3 months.
B. Breakthrough bleeding is treated with conjugated estrogen 1.25 mg or estradiol 2 mg daily for 7d. Continue to take the contraceptive pills.
C. Exclude pregnancy if breakthrough bleeding occurs, especially if missed pills, breast tenderness, nausea, or vomiting.

VIII. Commonly Used Oral Contraceptive Pills
A. Monophasic
   1. **21/7 Regimen (21 days of combined progestin and estrogen and 7 days of placebo)**
      a) Alesse, Levlite, Aviane, Lessina, Lutera—Levonorgestrel 0.1/ethinyl estradiol 20
      b) Loestrin 21 1/20, Loestrin Fe 1/20, Microgestin Fe 1/20, Junel Fe 1/20— Norethindrone acetate 1/ethinyl estradiol 20
      c) Yasmin, Ocella —Drospirenone 3/ethinyl estradiol 30
      d) Nordette, Levlen, Levora —Levonorgestrel 0.15/ethinyl estradiol 30
      e) Loestrin 21 1.5/30, Loestrin FE 1.5/30, Microgestin FE 1.5/30, Junel 1.5/30—Norethindrone acetate 1.5/ethinyl estradiol 30
      f) Desogen, Ortho-Cept, Apri —Desogestrel 0.15/ethinyl estradiol 30
      g) Cryselle, Lo Ovral, Low-Ogestrel —Norgestrel 0.3/ethinyl estradiol 30
      h) Ovcon 35, Femcon Fe (chewable) —Norethindrone 0.4/ethinyl estradiol 35
      i) Modicon, Brevicon, Necon 0.5/35, Nelova 0.5/35, Nortrel 0.5/35— Norethindrone 0.5/ethinyl estradiol 35
      j) Demulen 1/35, Zovia 1/35E, Kelnor 1/35 —Ethynodiol 1/ethinyl estradiol 35
      k) Previfem —Norgestimate 0.18/ethinyl estradiol 35
      l) OrthoCyclen, MonoNessa —Norgestimate 0.25/ethinyl estradiol 35
      m) Ortho-Novum 1/35, Norinyl 1/35, Necon 1/35, Nelova 1/35 — Norethindrone 1/ethinyl estradiol 35
      n) Ovcon 50 —Norethindrone 1/ethinyl estradiol 50
      o) Demulen 1/50, Zovia 1/50 E —Ethynodiol diacetate 1/ethinyl estradiol 50
      p) Ortho-Novum 1/50, Norinyl 1/50, Necon 1/50, Nelova 1/50 — Norethindrone 1/ mestranol 50
      q) Ovral, Ogestrel —Norgestrel 0.5/ethinyl estradiol 50
   2. **24/4 Regimen**
      a) Lo Loestrin Fe —Norethindrone acetate 1/ethinyl estradiol 10 for 24 tabs, 2 ethinyl estradiol tabs, 2 iron tabs
      b) Loestrin 24 Fe —norethindrone acetate 1/ethinyl estradiol 20 for 24 tabs, 4 iron tabs
      c) Yaz —Drospirenone 3/ethinyl estradiol 20
      d) Beyaz —Yaz+folate calcium 0.451 mg
      e) Generess Fe —Norethindrone 0.8/ethinyl estradiol 25
   3. **Biphasic**
      a) OrthoNovum 10/11, Necon 10/11 —Norethindrone/ethinyl estradiol, 0.5/35 for 10d, 1/35 for 11 days
      b) Mircette, Kariva —Desogestrel/ethinyl estradiol, 0.15/20 for 21 days, placebo for 2d, estradiol for 5 days

IX. Triphasic

A. Natazia (24/4 regimen; 1 mg of E2 = 0.76mg of E2) —E2 valerate/dienogest, 3/0 for 2 days, 2/2 for 5 days, 2/3 for 17 days

B. Estrostep FE, Tilia Fe, TriLegest Fe —Norethindrone acetate/ethinyl estradiol, 1/20 for 5 days, 1/30 for 7 days, 1/35 for 9 days

C. Ortho Tri-Cyclen Lo —Norgestimate/ethinyl estradiol, 0.18/25 for 7 days, 0.215/25 for 7 days, 0.25/25 for 7 days

D. Cyclessa, Velivet —Desogestrel/ethinyl estradiol, 0.1/25 for 7 days, 0.125/25 for 7 days, 0.150 /25 for 7 days

E. Triphasil, Enpresse, Trilevlen —Levonorgestrel/ethinyl estradiol, 0.05/30 for 6 days, 0.075/40 for 5 days, 0.125/30 for 10 days

F. Tri-Norinyl, Aranelle —Norethindrone/ethinyl estradiol, 0.5/35 for 7d, 1/35 for 9d, 0.5/35 for 5d

G. Ortho Tri-Cyclen, TriNessa, Tri-Sprintec —Norgestimate/ethinyl estradiol, 0.18/35 for 7 days, 0.215/35 for 7 days, 0.25/35 for 7 days

H. OrthoNovum 7/7/7, Necon 7/7/7 —Norethindrone/ethinyl estradiol, 0.5/35 for 7 days, 0.75/35 for 7 days, 1/35 for 7 days

X. Extended or Continuous Regimens

A. Seasonale, Jolessa (84 active tabs + 7 placebo) —Levonorgestrel 0.15/ethinyl estradiol 30 for 84 days

B. Seasonique: 84 active tabs + 7 ethinyl estradiol (10 ug) — Levonorgestrel 0.15/ethinyl estradiol 30 for 84 days, 0.1 ethinyl estradiol for 7 days

C. Lybrel —Levonorgestrel 90 µg/ethinyl estradiol 20 daily (no scheduled menses)

XI. Progestin-Only Oral Contraceptives

A. Micronor, Errin, Nor-QD —Norethindrone 350 µg

B. Ovrette —Norgestrel 75 µg

XII. Emergency Contraception

A. **Levonorgestrel (Plan B)**
   1. Regimens: Plan B (levonorgestrel 0.75 mg): 1 tab po q12h for 2 or 2 tabs po for 1; Plan B One-Step (LNG 1.5 mg): 1 tab po for 1. There is no difference in efficacy or side effects
   2. Emergency contraception is available over-the-counter for patients ≥17 years age. A prescription is required if less than 17 years.
   3. Emergency contraception is effective for 5 days after unprotected intercourse.
   4. Pregnancy test is done if menses are delayed by more than one week.

B. **Ulipristal (Ella)**
   1. Ella is a selective progesterone receptor modulator, which suppresses endometrial growth and prevents implantation of the zygote.
   2. Dosage 30 mg po. Ella is a more effective than levonorgestrel when given with 120 hours (5 days) after unprotected intercourse.
   3. Ulipristal may increase the cycle length by delaying the onset of menses.

C. **Intrauterine System Emergency Contraception**
   1. When inserted up to 5 days, the copper intrauterine system is the most effective method for postcoital contraception.

XIII. Transdermal Patch and Vaginal Ring deliver daily combined estrogen and progesterone.

A. **Ortho Evra Patch**
   1. Ortho Evra is given as 1 patch each week for 3 weeks; 1 week patch-free. The patch is applied to the buttock, lower abdomen, upper outer arm, or upper torso excluding breasts. Do not reapply the patch to the same site.
   2. Daily dose of 150 µg norelgestromin and 20 µg ethinyl estradiol.

3. The patch has an increased failure rate in women weighing >90 kg (198 lbs).
4. Ortho Evra has an increased risk of venous thromboembolism compared to OCs.

B. **NuvaRing**
1. The NuvaRing is self-inserted into the vagina for 3 weeks; 1 week free permits withdrawal bleeding
2. The NuvaRing releases 15 µg of ethinyl estradiol and 120-µg of etonogestrel per day. The NuvaRing delivers the lowest estrogen level of the combined hormonal contraceptives.

XIV. **Injectable Hormone and Implant**
A. **Medroxyprogesterone Acetate**
1. Depo-Provera (DMPA) is administered as 150 mg IM q 12–14 weeks
2. Depo-SubQ Provera 104: 104 mg SC injection q12-14 weeks. Can be self-injected subcutaneously.
3. **Indications:** Medroxyprogesterone acetate is ideal for women with no desire for a rapid return to fertility (>1 year), estrogen-free contraception, breastfeeding, seizures, sickle cell disease, or mental retardation.
4. **Relative contraindications** to MPA include cerebral and cardiovascular disease, systolic BP ≥160 mm Hg or diastolic BP ≥100 mmHg, liver tumors, diabetic vascular disease, and systemic lupus erythematosus with positive antiphospholipid antibodies.

B. **Side Effects**
1. Irregular bleeding develops in 70% during first year. 80% are amenorrheic after 5 years of use. Treatment of irregular bleeding is NSAIDs or 1.25 mg of conjugated estrogen or 2 mg of estradiol qd for 7days
2. Medroxy progesterone acetate temporarily decreases bone mineral density due to suppression of estradiol. DEXA scans are not needed.
3. Weight gain is associated with intramuscular DMPA.

C. **Implanon (etonogestrel implant 68 mg)**
1. Implanon is a single-rod implant, which is placed under the skin on the inner, upper arm.
2. Implanon releases 30–50 mcg of etonogestrel daily and is effective for 3 years.
3. Implanon is the most effective birth control method with a failure rate of 0.05%.
4. Most common side effect is irregular bleeding.

XV. **Intrauterine Systems**
A. **Mechanisms of Action**: Intrauterine systems prevent fertilization because of a foreign body effect and intrauterine inflammatory reaction. Destruction of the fertilized ovum may also be caused by the IUS.
B. **Types of intrauterine systems**
1. **Copper intrauterine system TCu-380A (Paraguard)**
   a) Paraguard is approved for 10 years and is effective for 12 years. The patient continues to have normal periods
   b) Paraguard is associated with increased menstrual bleeding of up to 55% with intermenstrual spotting, and dysmenorrhea
   c) The discontinuation rate is 9.7% because of menorrhagia and dysmenorrhea
2. **Levonorgestrel intrauterine system (Mirena)**
   a) Mirena is approved for 5 years and is effective for up to 7 years. Levonorgestrel reduces menstrual bleeding; 50% have amenorrhea in 2 years.
   b) Prolonged irregular bleeding after the initial insertion may occur. Ovulation occurs in about 60% of women.

C. **Intrauterine System Contraindications**
1. Pelvic inflammatory disease, suspected pregnancy, uterine anomalies, and uterine cavity distortion.
2. The progesterone IUS is contraindicated in breast cancer.

D. **Intrauterine System Insertion**
1. Sexually transmitted disease screening and intrauterine system insertion can be done at same time in high-risk patients.
2. Intrauterine systems can be inserted any time during the menstrual cycle after a negative pregnancy test. Backup contraception is needed for 1 week after insertion of the levonorgestrel intrauterine system.
3. **Uterine perforation** can occur during intrauterine system insertion due to cervical stenosis, and anteverted or retroverted uterus.
4. Insertion of an IUS may cause a vasovagal response with nausea, syncope or presyncope, bradycardia, and hypotension. May give atropine 0.5 mg IM or IV for severe reactions.

XVI. **Sterilization**
A. Female and male sterilization is the most frequent contraceptive method among married couples. 27% of fertile women have sterilizations and 9.2% of women rely on vasectomies.

B. **Hysteroscopic Tubal Occlusion**
1. Essure is a metal and polymer micro-insert with a low risk of pregnancy of 0.1%.
2. Contraindications: pregnancy is within 6 weeks, active or recent pelvic inflammatory disease, uterine or tubal pathology, and allergy to contrast.
3. Endometrial thinning is achieved with progestin for 2 weeks before the procedure to facilitate visualization of tubal ostia.
4. Distension media is normal saline
5. Complications: uterine or tubal perforation (1%), device expulsion (1%), unsuccessful or unilateral insertion (6%), failed tubal occlusion at 3 months (3.5%), pelvic pain, and infection.
6. HSG is required to confirm bilateral tubal blockage at 3 months after the procedure.

Periodic Health Assessment

I. **Screening, Evaluation, and Counseling**
A. Counsel on contraception, diet, exercise, and weight. Folic acid 0.4 mg/day before age 50. Breast self-exam.
B. The first gynecologic visit should be at age 13–15, followed by annual visits. Internal pelvic exams are not needed at age 13–18. Perform pelvic exam if sexually active, abnormal bleeding, pelvic pain, or vaginitis.
C. **Chlamydia and Gonorrhea.** Screen for Chlamydia and gonorrhea if age ≤25 and sexually active.
D. **HIV Screening.** HIV testing for women age 19–64 years.
E. **Mammogram.** Mammogram every 1–2 years beginning at age 40, and then yearly after age 50 year.
F. **Colon Cancer**
1. Colon cancer screening should begin at age 50 years.
2. Colonoscopy every 10 years
G. **Thyroid Diseases.** TSH every 5 years, beginning at age 50 years
H. **Lipid Profile.** Fasting lipid profile every 5 years, beginning at age 45 year.
I. **Diabetes.** Fasting glucose every 3 years, beginning at age 45 years
J. **Osteoporosis.** DEXA testing is indicated for all women ≥ 65 years,

every 2 years. Early testing should be performed for women with risk factors for osteoporosis

II. Pelvic Examination

A. Speculum Examination

1. Lubricate the blades with gel before insertion. Lubricant does not interfere with cervical culture and cytology.
2. Insert the speculum in a 45^0 angle toward rectum. Apply pressure posteriorly because of the distensibility of posterior vaginal wall.

B. Bimanual Examination

1. Insert two fingers into the posterior fornix and elevate the uterus anteriorly toward the hand on the abdomen.
2. Move vaginal fingers deeply into lateral fornix to palpate the adnexa.

C. Rectovaginal Examination

1. A rectovaginal exam is indicated if the patient has a malignancy, endometriosis, pelvic prolapse, or a retroverted uterus.
2. Rectovaginal exam is performed by inserting well-lubricated middle finger into the rectum first, then insert the index finger into the vagina.

III. Breast Examinations

A. The breast examination is best conducted 7–10 days after the onset of menses for premenopausal women.

B. Breast examination includes inspection and palpation of breast in sitting and supine positions.

IV. HPV Vaccination

A. Routine vaccination is recommended at 11–12 years. HPV vaccines are not recommended for pregnant women.

V. Gardasil

A. Recombinant quadrivalent HPV vaccine prevents infection by HPV 6, 11, 16, and 18. HPV 6 and 11 cause about 90% of genital warts; HPV 16 and 18 cause 70% of cervical cancers.

B. Gardasil is approved for use in females and males aged 9–26 years.

C. Three IM injections are given at 0, 2, and 6 months.

VI. Cervarix

A. Cervarix is a recombinant bivalent HPV vaccine for prevention of HPV 16 and 18 infection.

B. Cervarix is approved for use in females, aged 10 to 25 years.

C. Cervarix is administered in three doses at 0, 1, and 6 month intervals.

VII. Gynecological Care for Women with HIV Infection

A. HIV Transmission and Prevention

1. 72% of HIV transmission among women results from sexual intercourse.
2. Screen HIV infection in women aged 19–64.

B. Cervical Cancer Screening in HIV-Infected Women

1. HIV-infected women are at high risk of HPV infection and CIN. Cervical cytology should be completed twice in the first year after diagnosis of HIV infection and then annually.
2. HPV testing is not advised for triaging HIV-infected women with abnormal cytology or for follow-up after treatment for CIN.
3. For ASC-US or higher, perform colposcopy.
4. CIN 1 should be followed by cervical cytology after 6 and 12 months.
5. CIN 2 or CIN 3 is managed with ablation or excision if the woman is 21 years and older. In the first year after treatment, follow-up is done with cervical cytology at 6-month intervals.

C. **Birth Control**
   1. Women taking HAART may use copper or levonorgestrel intrauterine system, Depo-Provera, and progesterone implants.
   2. Ritonavir-boosted protease inhibitors and non-nucleoside reverse transcriptase inhibitors reduce efficacy of hormonal contraception. Women taking ART should avoid oral contraceptives.
   3. If pregnancy is desired, maximum suppression of viral load is needed before conception. Avoid efavirenz because of CNS and neural tube defects.

D. **Vaccination**
   1. HIV-infected women should receive routine vaccinations. Live vaccines are contraindicated.

Breast Cancer Screening

I. **Breast Cancer Risk Assessment**
   A. Breast cancer is the most frequently diagnosed cancer. Breast cancer is second leading cause of death from cancer in American women. The lifetime risk of breast cancer is 12% or 1 in 8 women.

II. **Clinical Risk Factors and Relative Risks**
   A. **Reproductive hormonal factors**
      1. Early menarche: RR 1.1
      2. Menopause after 51 years: RR 1.1
      3. Nulliparity: RR 1.1
      4. First birth after age 35 years: RR 1.5
      5. Menopausal hormone replacement therapy: RR 1.31
      6. Breastfeeding >1 year: RR 0.7 (RR <1 is protective against breast cancer)
      7. Menopause before age 40 years: RR 0.5
   B. **Genetic factors**
      1. Family history of one first-degree relative with breast cancer: RR 2.0
      2. Family history of two first-degree relatives with breast cancer: RR 6.9
      3. BRCA gene mutation: 40–80% lifetime risk

III. **Breast Cancer Screening Guidelines**
   A. **ACOG Guidelines on Breast Cancer Screening**
      1. Women age 40 or older should be offered screening mammogram annually.
      2. Clinical breast exam for women age ≥40 years, perform annually. For women age 20–39 years, perform CBE every 1 to 3 years.
   B. **USPSTF Recommendations**
      1. Biennial screening mammography at age 50 to 74
      2. The current evidence is inadequate to assess the benefits of screening women 75 years or older.
      3. Recommends against teaching BSE.
      4. Evidence is inadequate to assess the additional benefits of CBE in women 40 years or older.
   C. **Breast Cancer Susceptibility Genes**
      1. BRCA1 and BRCA2 are cancer suppressor genes.
      2. BRCA1 mutations account for half of all inherited breast cancers and 90% of hereditary ovarian cancers. BRCA2 mutations account for 40% of inherited breast cancers and 5% of hereditary ovarian cancers.
      3. Women with a BRCA 1 or a BRCA 2 mutations have life-time risk of breast cancer of 56–84%.

4. Women with a BRCA 1 mutations have a 36–63% life-time risk of ovarian cancer. With BRCA 2 mutation, the life-time risk of ovarian cancer is 10–27%.

D. **USPSTF Criteria for Genetic Risk Assessment and BRCA Testing**
1. **Any woman with family history of the following**
   a) Two first-degree relatives with breast cancer, at least 1 of whom diagnosed at ≤50 years
   b) Three or more first- or second-degree relatives with breast cancer diagnosed at any age
   c) A combination of both breast and ovarian cancer among first- or second-degree relatives
   d) A first-degree relative with bilateral breast cancer
   e) A combination of 2 or more first- or second-degree relatives with ovarian cancer
   f) A first- or second-degree relatives with both breast and ovarian cancer
   g) A male relative with breast cancer

IV. Screening Mammography

A. Sensitivity of mammography is 95%. Specificity of mammography is 97%.
B. Dense breast and young age have a decreased sensitivity and specificity of mammography and increase false-negative rate and false positive rate.
C. Malignancy appears as clusters of small calcifications. Masses appear as an area of radiodensity or breast parenchymal distortion or skin thickening and edema.

Breast Diseases

I. Benign Breast Diseases

A. Mastalgia

1. Mastalgia accounts for up to 50% of breast-related complaints.
2. Two-thirds of women with mastalgia have cyclic breast pain, which starts in the luteal phase and resolves with menses. Mastalgia is usually bilateral and associated with fibrocystic changes.
3. A breast examination and ultrasound or mammogram should be performed. Pregnancy should be excluded.

B. Treatment

1. Cancer-related pain is usually unilateral, noncyclic, and progressive. Breast pain is not a common presentation of early-stage breast cancer.
2. Treatment of mastalgia is a fitted brassiere and avoidance of cigarettes, caffeine, and stress.
3. NSAIDs
4. Low-dose oral contraceptives in a continuous regimen.
5. Tamoxifen 10 to 20 mg po qd
6. Bromocriptine 2.5 mg po 2 times a day, increase as tolerated

C. Breast Cysts

1. Breast cysts are usually asymptomatic
2. Ultrasound is performed if the patient is ≤30 years age. Ultrasound and mammogram are performed if the patient is >30 years age.
3. Observe if ultrasound indicates simple cyst. If aspiration is performed, fluid should be discarded if it is clear, yellow or green. Bloody fluid should be evaluated for cytology.
4. Perform biopsy if the cyst has a thick wall, septation or a solid component.

D. **Fibroadenoma**
1. Fibroadenoma is the most common benign tumor in women of age 20–35 years of age.
2. The fibroadenomas are mobile, nontender, firm, and solitary.
3. Biopsy is indicated to confirm the diagnosis.
4. Treatment: Observation of fibroadenomas is advised if there is no growth. Excise the fibroadenoma if preferred by the patient.

E. **Nipple Discharge**
1. Nipple discharge is usually benign in women less than 60 years of age. The discharge can be watery, serous, green, or bloody.
2. Signs of non-neoplastic discharges galactorrhea, discharge from manipulation of the breast, and bilateral or multiductal discharge.
3. Pathologic discharges are spontaneous, single duct, and bloody or serous. Causes of pathologic discharge include intraductal papilloma, ductal ectasia, and cancer
4. **Breast examination.** Apply pressure to express discharge from the nipples, and evaluate unilaterality or bilaterality, uniductality or multiductality, and color of the discharge.
5. Treatment: Image with ultrasound and mammogram. Ductogram and terminal duct excision may be performed.

F. **Galactorrhea**
1. Galactorrhea is a milky discharge from multiple ducts in nonlactating women. Galactorrhea is visible as multiple fat droplets under microscopy.
2. **Etiology:** Galactorrhea can be idiopathic, or caused by breast stimulation, OCs, hypothyroidism, pituitary tumors, hyperprolactinemia, phenothiazine, reserpine, amphetamine, opiates, diazepam, methyldopa, TCAs, and butyrophenones.
3. Evaluation: Measure TSH and prolactin. Pituitary MRI is done if prolactin is elevated.

II. **Evaluation of Breast Mass**
   A. **Clinical Breast Examination:** Signs of breast cancer include single lesions with hard, immobile, and irregular borders
   B. **Breast ultrasound** is useful for young women and pregnant or lactating women. Ultrasound is used to guide biopsy. Breast ultrasound differentiates solid from cystic lesions
   C. **Mammogram**
   1. Diagnostic mammogram is performed for breast symptoms and abnormal breast examinations.
   2. Mammogram is less sensitive in young women because of high breast density
   D. **Fine-Needle Aspiration**
   1. Fine-needle aspiration is used for palpable breast masses to obtain cells for cytologic testing.
   2. **Triple-Test:** includes clinical breast exam, breast imaging, and FNA cytology.
      a) Accuracy of FNAB is 100% if all three tests are concordant.
      b) If all three parts of triple test are benign, observation with serial follow-up or excision are recommended in premenopausal women.
      c) In postmenopausal women, a new dominant mass should be excised after obtaining a tissue diagnosis with needle biopsy.
   E. **Core Needle Biopsy**
   1. Core needle biopsy provides a specimen for histopathologic diagnosis.
   2. Core needle biopsy can be preformed under ultrasound or X-ray. Sensitivity and specificity of stereotactic CNB is 85-100%.

F. **Mammographically Localized Biopsy**
  1. Mammographically localized biopsy should only be used when FNA and CNB are not possible or when results of needle biopsy indicate a need for operative biopsy.
  2. A needle or wire is placed at the site of suspected abnormality in the mammography suite. Open biopsy excises the abnormality. Radiograph is performed on the surgical specimen.

III. **Treatment of Breast Cancer**
  A. **Two-step approach:** (1) outpatient biopsy; (2) definitive treatment with histologic diagnosis
  B. **Sentinel Lymph Node Biopsy**
    1. Sentinel lymph node biopsy is used in early breast cancer without palpable lymph node metastases.
    2. Sentinel lymph node biopsy removes 2–3 sentinel lymph nodes for histological exam. If SLN is negative, no axillary dissection is performed.
    3. Sentinel lymph node biopsy avoids lymphedema, paresthesias, and pain, caused by axillary node dissection.
  C. **Breast Conserving Surgery**. The combination of segmental mastectomy, axillary lymph node dissection and postoperative radiation are as effective as mastectomy for stage 1 and stage 2 cancers.
  D. **Adjuvant Chemotherapy**
    1. Patients with >10% of risk for systemic disease are candidates for chemotherapy.
    2. In estrogen receptor positive, lymph node negative patients, multigene assays on tumor specimens are used to assess risk of distant metastasis and benefit of chemotherapy.
  E. **Chemotherapy Regimens for Breast Cancer**
    1. Docetaxel and cyclophosphamide
    2. Docetaxel, doxorubicin, and cyclophosphamide
    3. Doxorubicin, cyclophosphamide, and paclitaxel
    4. Doxorubicin and cyclophosphamide
  F. **Adjuvant Hormonal Therapy**
    1. **Selective Estrogen Receptor Modulators**
    2. *Tamoxifen*
      a) Tamoxifen is an estrogen antagonist and agonist, which blocks endogenous estrogen in the breast. Tamoxifen has estrogenic effects in the uterus, bones, and liver.
      b) Tamoxifen decreases breast cancer recurrence by 50% and reduces mortality by 31% in women with positive estrogen receptors.
      c) Tamoxifen increases the risk of endometrial cancer, thromboembolism, endometrial polyps, and hot flashes.
    3. *Raloxifene*
      a) Raloxifene has estrogen antagonist effects on the breast and uterus and estrogenic effects on the bone and lipids.
      b) Raloxifene is used in high risk patients for breast cancer prevention. Raloxifene is not used for breast cancer adjuvant therapy.
      c) Raloxifene is less effective than tamoxifen in preventing invasive breast cancer.
      d) Raloxifene has a lower risk of endometrial cancer than tamoxifen.
      e) Raloxifene increases risk of thromboembolism; however, the risk is less than for tamoxifen
      f) Raloxifene is used to prevent and treat osteoporosis.

4. *Aromatase Inhibitors*
   a) Aromatase inhibitors include anastrozole (Arimidex), letrozole (Femara), and exemestane (Aromasin).
   b) Aromatase inhibitors have antiestrogenic effects and reduce endogenous estrogen by 95% by preventing peripheral conversion of androgens to estrogens.
   c) Aromatase inhibitors are used for postmenopausal women with positive hormone receptors.
   d) Aromatase inhibitors are associated with increased risk of osteoporosis and fracture. Aromatase inhibitors have a lower risk of endometrial cancer, cerebrovascular events, venous thromboemboli and hot flushes than tamoxifen.

G. **Adjuvant Biologic Therapy –Trastuzumab (Herceptin)**
   1. Herceptin decreases recurrence and mortality by 50% and 33% in women with over-expression of HER2/neu or amplification of HER2 gene.
   2. Trastuzumab can be given with chemotherapy or after chemotherapy. Trastuzumab may not be given concurrently with anthracyclines because of the risk of CHF.

Cervical Cancer Screening

I. **Cervical Cancer Screening**
   A. **Cervical cytology (Pap):** includes conventional and liquid-based Pap tests.
   B. **HPV testing** for high-risk cervical cancer-causing HPV types includes HPV type 16 and 18 . Other high-risk types include type 31, 33, 35, 39, 45, 51, 52, and 58.

II. **Diagnosis of Preinvasive Lesions**
   A. Colposcopy and biopsy. Colposcopy differentiates malignant and premalignant epithelium based on contour, color, and vascular pattern. Abnormal areas of the cervix are biopsied.
   B. Preinvasive lesions are CIN1, CIN2, CIN3, or CIN 2–3.

III. **Treatment of Preinvasive Lesions**
   A. **Excisional procedures:** LEEP or cold knife cone
   B. **Ablative procedures** include cryotherapy, laser ablation, or fulguration

IV. **Cervical Cytology**
   A. **Squamous Cell Abnormalities**
      1. Atypical squamous cells (ASC)
         a) Of undetermined significance (ASC-US)
         b) Cannot exclude HSIL (ASC-H)
      2. Low-grade squamous intraepithelial lesions (LSIL). Encompassing human papillomavirus (HPV), mild dysplasia and cervical intraepithelial neoplasia (CIN1)
      3. High-grade squamous intraepithelial lesions (HSIL). Encompassing moderate and severe dysplasia, carcinoma in situ, CIN 2, and CIN 3
      4. Squamous cell carcinoma
   B. **Glandular Cell Abnormalities**
      1. Atypical glandular cells (AGC): specify endocervical, endometrial, or not otherwise specified (NOS)
      2. Atypical endocervical cells, favor neoplastic (specify endocervical or NOS)
      3. Endocervical adenocarcinoma in situ (AIS)
      4. Adenocarcinoma

V. ACOG Recommendations for Cervical Cytology Screening

   A. **Age to start screening:** Begin screening at age 21. Women less than 21 years should not be screened.

   B. **Age 21–29**: Screening with cytology every 3 years. Co-testing should not be performed.

   C. **Age 30–65**: Screening with HPV and cytology co-testing every 5 years

   D. **ASC-US/ HPV co-testing negative**: Routine screening every 5 years due to very low risk of CIN 3.

   E. **Co-testing Negative cytology/ positive HPV**
      1. Repeat cotesting in 12 months. If repeat test LSIL or HPV still positive, proceed to colposcopy OR
      2. Immediate HPV genotyping for HPV 16/18. If positive, proceed to colposcopy. If negative, cotest in 12 months. If cotest shows positive HPV or LSIL, perform colposcopy.

   F. **Screening after total hysterectomy**: If no history of CIN 2 or higher, cytology and HPV testing should be discontinued. If history of CIN 2 or higher, screen with cytology for 20 years.

   G. **History of CIN 2, 3 or adenocarcinoma in situ**: Routine age-based screening for 20 years after initial post-treatment surveillance.

   H. **Age to stop screening**: Age 65 with no history of CIN 2 or higher and 3 consecutive negative cytology or 2 consecutive negative co-tests, with most recent test done in the last 5 years.

VI. Treatment of Abnormal Cytology in Adolescents

   A. **ASC-US, LSIL, and CIN 1:** Repeat cytology at 12-month intervals for 2 years. Perform colposcopy if abnormality persists for 2 years.

   B. **HSIL and ASC-H:** Perform colposcopy. If CIN 2–3, perform colposcopy and cytology at 6-month intervals for 2 years, provided that ECC is negative. Diagnostic excisional procedure if HSIL persists at 24 months.

   C. **CIN 3:** should be treated with cryotherapy, laser, and LEEP.

VII. Cervical Cancer Screening in Women with HIV: Cervical cytology should be performed two times in the first year and then annually.

VIII. Benign Endometrial Cells Found in Cervical Cytology

   A. Benign endometrial cells on Pap test do not require evaluation in asymptomatic premenopausal women.

   B. Perform endometrial biopsy in postmenopausal women or premenopausal women with abnormal uterine bleeding, chronic anovulation, or obesity.

IX. HPV Testing

   A. HPV screening is only used in women ≥30 years of age.

   B. HPV genotyping is useful to triage the patient with high-risk HPV and negative cytology.

X. Colposcopy

   A. Normal squamous epithelium does not stain with acetic acid. Normal squamous epithelium stains brown with iodine

   B. The transformation zone is located between the original and current squamocolumnar junctions squamous metaplasia. CIN, and cervical cancer develop in the transformation zone. Major cellular changes occur during puberty and the first pregnancy. After menopause, the SCJ is located in the endocervix.

   C. Metaplasia appears as smooth areas with fine, uniform sized vessels. Meta plasia demonstrates mild acetowhite change and negative Lugol's iodine stain.

XI. Colposcopic Terminology of the International Federation for Cervical Pathology and Colposcopy
   A. **General Assessment**
      1. Adequate or insufficient;
      2. Squamocolumnar junction visibility: completely visible, partially visible, not visible;
      3. Transformation zone types 1, 2, or 3
   B. **Normal Findings**
      1. Original squamous epithelium is mature, atrophic;
      2. Columnar epithelium, ectopy/ectropion;
      3. Metaplastic squamous epithelium, nabothian cysts, crypt (gland) openings;
      4. Deciduosis in pregnancy
   C. **Abnormal Colposcopic Findings**
      1. Location of the lesion: inside or outside of the transformation zone. Location by the clock position
      2. Size of the lesion: number of cervical quadrants covered by the lesions
      3. Size of the lesion as percentage of cervix
      4. *Grade 1 (minor):* fine mosaic. Fine punctation. Thin acetowhite epithelium. Irregular, border
      5. *Grade 2 (major):* sharp border. Inner border sign. Ridge sign. Dense acetowhite epithelium. Coarse mosaic. Coarse punctation. Rapid acetowhitening. Cuffed crypt openings
      6. *Nonspecific:* leukoplakia (keratosis, hyperkeratosis), erosion; Lugol's staining
   D. **Suspicious for invasion**
      1. Atypical vessels
      2. Fragile vessels, irregular surface, exophytosis, necrosis, ulceration, tumor or neoplasm
   E. **Miscellaneous findings**
      1. Congenital transformation zone, condyloma, polyps, inflammation, stenosis, congenital anomaly, endometriosis
XII. Indications for Treatment of Cervical Intraepithelial Neoplasia
   A. CIN 2–3
   B. HSIL
   C. Lesion persists ≥2 years in CIN 1 preceded by ASC-US, ASC-H or LSIL:
      1. Diagnostic excisional procedures if colposcopy is unsatisfactory, ECC positive for CIN, or history of previous treatment.
      2. Continued follow-up is also acceptable.
   D. CIN 1 preceded by HSIL or AGC-NOS: Follow-up with colposcopy and cytology at 6-month intervals for 1 year.
XIII. Indications for Hysterectomy for CIN
   A. Hysterectomy may be considered as an alternative option to diagnostic excision in the following situations:
      1. Recurrent or persistent CIN 2–3
      2. CIN 2–3 lesion is identified at the margins of an excisional specimen or in the endocervical canal.
         a) Cytology and endocervical sampling at 4–6 months is the recommended management.
         b) Hysterectomy is acceptable if repeat diagnostic excisional procedure is not possible.

Vaginitis

Vaginitis presents with discharge, itching, burning, odor, dysuria and dyspareunia. Vulvar erythema, edema, and excoriation is common.

I. Normal Vaginal Discharge
A. Normal vaginal discharge is white, thin, and floccular.
B. Vaginal pH is normally <4.5.
C. Epithelial cells and lactobacilli are normally visible on microscopy.

II. Bacterial Vaginosis
A. Bacterial vaginosis is the most common cause of abnormal discharge and malodor. Bacterial vaginosis is asymptomatic in 50%.
B. The normal hydrogen peroxide producing Lactobacillus are replaced by an overgrowth of anaerobic bacteria, such as Prevotella, Mobiluncus, Gardnerella vaginalis, and Mycoplasma hominis.
C. Microscopy demonstrates clue cells, which are epithelial cells covered with coccobacilli.

III. Diagnosis
A. **Point-of-care testing** kits are used for the diagnosis of bacterial vaginosis if wet prep is unavailable.
B. Bacterial Vaginosis is diagnosed by 3 out of the following:
1. A homogeneous, thin, white, noninflammatory discharge
2. Clue cells on microscopy
3. A pH of vaginal fluid >4.5
4. "Whiff" test: A fishy odor of vaginal discharge after addition of 10% KOH

IV. Treatment
A. Women with symptoms should be treated. Incidental bacterial vaginosis found on cervical cytology does not require treatment.
B. Routine treatment of sex partner is not advised.

V. Treatment of Bacterial Vaginosis
A. Metronidazole (Flagyl) 500 mg PO 2 times a day for 7 days. Avoid alcohol during and after treatment for 3 days if using metronidazole and tinidazole.
or
B. Metronidazole (Metrogel) gel 0.75% (Metrogel), 1 applicator (5 g) vaginally, qd for 5 days, or
C. Clindamycin cream 2%, 1 applicator (5 g) vaginally qhs for 7 days
D. **Alternative Regimens**
1. Tinidazole (Tindamax) 2 g PO qd for 3 days; avoid alcohol or
2. Tinidazole (Tindamax) 1 g PO qd for 5 days; avoid alcohol or
3. Two percent extended-release clindamycin cream (Clindesse), 1 applicator vaginally. Metronidazole, 750 mg extended-release tablets, qd for 7 days
4. Multiple recurrence after treatment is managed with metronidazole gel twice weekly for 4–6 months.
E. **Bacterial Vaginosis in Pregnancy**
1. Bacterial vaginosis is associated with premature rupture of membranes, preterm labor, intraamniotic infection, and endometritis. Screening for bacterial vaginosis is not advised.
2. Pregnant women with symptoms of bacterial vaginosis should be treated with Metronidazole (Flagyl) 500 mg PO 2 times a day for 7 days or 250 mg tid for 7 days or clindamycin 300 mg 2 times a day for 7 days.

VI. Trichomoniasis

A. Trichomoniasis may be asymptomatic or cause a diffuse, malodorous, yellow-green discharge with vulvar irritation.

B. Trichomoniasis causes copious, frothy, yellow-to-green, malodorous discharge with a "strawberry" cervix and a fishy odor

C. **Diagnosis**

1. Point-of-care testing for trichomonas has sensitivity >83% and specificity >97%.

2. Wet prep demonstrates trichomonas and many WBC's in vaginal fluid.

3. Culture for T. vaginalis is highly sensitive and specific.

4. Cervical cytology finding of trichomonas should be confirmed with wet prep.

D. **Treatment**

1. Vaginal metronidazole gel is not advised for trichomoniasis because of minimal penetration into the paravaginal glands.

2. The patient's sex partner should be treated.

3. Metronidazole (Flagyl) 2 grams po or

4. Tinidazole (Tindamax) 2 grams PO

5. Metronidazole (Flagyl) 500 mg 2 times a day for 7 days is used for treatment failure after a single dose treatment.

E. **Trichomoniasis in Pregnancy**

1. Trichomoniasis is associated with premature rupture of membranes, preterm labor, and low birth weight.

2. Pregnant women with asymptomatic trichomoniasis should be treated with 2 g of metronidazole for 1.

VII. Vulvovaginal Candidiasis

A. Overgrowth of Candida albicans causes vulvovaginal candidiasis. Treatment of sexual partners is not advised.

B. Symptoms of candidiasis include vulvovaginal pruritus, vaginal soreness, dyspareunia, and abnormal discharge

C. Signs of vulvar erythema, edema, fissures, excoriations, and cottage-cheese-like discharge attached to the vaginal wall.

D. Wet prep with 10% KOH identifies pseudohyphae.

E. Culture can confirm diagnosis for recurrent or persistent candidiasis.

F. **Uncomplicated Vulvovaginal Candidiasis**

1. **Prescription Agents**

a) Butoconazole 2% cream, 5 g vaginally for 1

b) Terconazole 0.4% cream 5 g vaginally for 7 days

c) Terconazole 0.8% cream 5 g vaginally for 3 days

d) Terconazole 80 mg vaginal suppository, 1 supp for 3 days

e) Oral regimen: fluconazole (Diflucan) 150 mg po for 1

G. **Treatment for Recurrent Vulvovaginal Candidiasis**

1. Topical therapy for 7–14 days

2. Fluconazole (Diflucan) 100 mg, 150 mg, or 200 mg po on day 1, 4, and 7

H. **Maintenance Regimens**

1. Fluconazole 100 mg, 150 mg, or 200 mg po weekly for 6 months

2. Vaginal clotrimazole 200 mg twice a week or 500 mg once a week.

I. **Treatment for Severe VVC or Immunosuppression**: Topical azole for 7–14 days or fluconazole given as two oral doses separated by 3 days.

J. **Treatment for Non-albican Vulvovaginitis**

1. Oral or topical azole for 7–14 days (not fluconazole)

2. If an azole is ineffective, give 600 mg of boric acid in a gelatin capsule vaginally for 2 weeks.

K. **Treatment of Vulvovaginal Candidiasis in Pregnancy**

1. Topical azole for 7 days.

Sexually Transmitted Diseases

I. **Sexually Transmitted Disease Reporting**
   A. Syphilis, gonorrhea, chlamydia, chancroid, and HIV/AIDS are reportable diseases.
II. **Chlamydia**
   A. Chlamydia is the most common sexually transmitted disease. Chlamydia infection is usually asymptomatic. Sexually active women ≤25 years old should be screened yearly.
   B. Chlamydia is diagnosed by urine or by swabs of the endocervix or vagina.
   C. **Treatment**
      1. Azithromycin (Zithromax) 1 g or
      2. Doxycycline 100 mg po 2 times a day for 7 days
      3. **Alternatives:** erythromycin base 500 mg 4 times a day for 7 days, erythromycin ethylsuccinate 800 mg po qid for 7 days, ofloxacin 300 mg 2 times a day for 7 days, or levofloxacin 500 mg po qd for 7days
      4. Retest in 3 months.
   D. **Chlamydia in Pregnancy**
      1. Retesting in the third trimester is advised for women less than 25 years or at increased risk for chlamydia.
      2. Azithromycin (Zithromax) 1 g for 1 or amoxicillin 500 mg po tid for 7 days
      3. Erythromycin base 500 mg qid for 7 days or 250 mg qid for 14 days. Erythromycin ethylsuccinate 800 mg qid for 7 days or 400 mg qid for 14 days
      4. Test-of-cure is advised in pregnancy, 3–4 weeks after treatment false positive result will occur because of uncleared chlamydial DNA if testing is done sooner.
III. **Gonorrhea**
   A. Gonorrhea is often asymptomatic and often coexists with Chlamydia. Screening women < 25 years old is advised. Endocervical, vaginal, or urine testing is diagnostic.
   B. **Recommended Treatment**
      1. Ceftriaxone (Rocephin) 250 mg IM PLUS
      2. Azithromycin (Zithromax) 1 g orally or doxycycline 100 mg orally twice daily for 7 days
   C. **Severe Cephalosporin Allergy:**
      1. Azithromycin (Zithromax) 2 g oral dose
      2. Test-of-cure in 1 week
IV. **Cervicitis**
   A. Cervicitis may be asymptomatic or may cause vaginal discharge, intermenstrual bleeding, and postcoital bleeding.
   B. **Diagnosis**
      1. Cervicitis causes a purulent or mucopurulent endocervical exudates
      2. Bleeding may be induced by passage of a cotton swab through the cervical os
      3. Test for Chlamydia and gonorrhea
   C. **Treatment**: Azithromycin (Zithromax) 1 g po; or doxycycline 100 mg po 2 times a day for 7 days
V. **Genital Herpes**
   A. Herpes is the most common cause of genital ulcers.
   B. HSV causes life-long recurrent infections with intermittent virus shedding. Genital herpes is usually due to HSV-2.

C. **Diagnosis**
1. HSV causes painful, multiple, vesicular or ulcerative genital lesions.
2. Viral culture of the lesions has a low sensitivity.
3. Type-specific serologic assay has a sensitivity of 98% and specificity of 96%.

D. **Treatment of First Episode**
1. Acyclovir (Zovirax) 400 mg po 3 times a day for 7–10 days. Famciclovir (Famvir) 250 mg po tid for 7–10 days. Valacyclovir (Valtrex) 1 g po 2 times a day for 7–10 days

E. **Recurrent Episode**
1. Acyclovir 800 mg 2 times a day for 5d. Acyclovir 800 mg tid for 2d. Famciclovir 125 mg 2 times a day for 5 days. Famciclovir 1,000 mg 2 times a day for 1 day. Famciclovir 500 mg, then 250 mg 2 times a day for 2 days. Valacyclovir 500 mg 2 times a day for 3 days, or valacyclovir 1 g qd for 5 days

F. **Severe Disease**
1. Disseminated infection, pneumonitis, hepatitis, or encephalitis.
2. Treatment: acyclovir 5–10 mg/kg IV q8h for 2–7 days or until improvement, followed by oral therapy for a total of at least 10-days.

G. **Suppressive Therapy**
1. Suppressive therapy decreases recurrences by 80% and decreases the risk for HSV-2 transmission to partners.
2. Acyclovir 400 mg 2 times a day; famciclovir (Famvir) 250 mg 2 times a day, valacyclovir 1 g qd, or valacyclovir (Valtrex) 500 mg qd.

VI. **Condyloma Acuminatum**
A. 90% of genital warts are due to HPV 6 or 11. Gardasil, a quadrivalent vaccine, can be used in females and males, 9–26 years to prevent genital warts.
B. Diagnosis is by visual examination.
C. Genital warts resolve spontaneously in 1 to 5 years in 90%.
D. **Treatment**
1. **Patient-Applied Regimens for External Genital Warts**
   a) Imiquimod 5% cream (Aldara) qhs 3 times/week up to 16 weeks or imiquimod 3.5% cream (Zyclara) daily for up to 8 weeks. Wash with soap and water 6–10h after application.
   b) Podofilox 0.5% solution or gel 2 times a day for 3 days.
   c) Sinecatechins (Veregen) 15% ointment 3 times daily for 16 weeks. Do not wash off. Effective in 77%.
2. **Physician-Applied Regimens**
   a) Cryotherapy with liquid nitrogen or cryoprobe. Repeat applications may be needed.
   b) Podophyllin resin 25% applied to each wart weekly. Limit application to less than 0.5 ml of podophyllin.
   c) Trichloroacetic acid or bichloroacetic acid 90% weekly.
   d) Surgical removal by scissors, shaving, curettage, or electrosurgery.

VII. **Molluscum Contagiosum**
A. Poxvirus infection is spread by sexual or close personal contact.
B. Molluscum contagiosum lesions are dome-shaped with a central umbilication.
C. **Treatment of Molluscum Contagiosum**
1. Often resolves spontaneously in immunocompetent patients.
2. Cryotherapy with liquid nitrogen, repeat in 2–3 weeks.
3. The curette is also effective

VIII. **Syphilis**
A. Syphilis is a systemic disease due to the spirochete, Treponema pallidum.

B. Nontreponemal tests, such as VDRL and RPR titers, reflect disease activity and become nonreactive after treatment. False-positive tests may be associated with other medical conditions.

C. Treponemal tests detect treponemal antibody with fluorescent treponemal antibody absorbed (FTA-ABS), T pallidum particle agglutination (TP-PA) or enzyme immunoassays. Treponemal tests remain positive after treatment.

D. A positive VDRL/RPR is automatically confirmed by treponemal syphilis IgG testing.

E. **Diagnosis**
   1. If nontreponemal and treponemal tests are positive and there is no history of treatment, the patient has active syphilis.
   2. If the patient was previously treated, the treponemal test usually remains reactive, but VDRL/RPR should become negative.
   3. Both tests can be falsely negative in 20% of primary syphilis. Darkfield microscopy or direct fluorescent antibody (DFA) can be used for diagnosis.

F. **Clinical Stage and Treatment**
   1. **Primary Syphilis**
      a) Painless ulcers or chancre at the site of infection. Darkfield exam and fluorescent antibody tests of exudates are diagnostic.
      b) Benzathine penicillin G 2.4 million units IM
   2. **Secondary Syphilis**
      a) Skin rash, mucocutaneous lesions, and lymphadenopathy
      b) Benzathine penicillin G 2.4 million units IM
   3. **Latent Syphilis**: Serologic tests are reactive, but signs and symptoms are absent
   4. *Early Latent*
      a) Latent syphilis is acquired within the preceding year
      b) The treatment of early latent syphilis is benzathine penicillin G 2.4 million units IM
   5. *Late Latent*
      a) Latent syphilis acquired for more than 1 year or latent syphilis of unknown duration
      b) Benzathine penicillin G 2.4 million units IM weekly for 3 weeks
   6. **Tertiary Syphilis**
      a) *Gumma and cardiovascular syphilis:* Benzathine penicillin G 2.4 million units IM weekly for 3 weeks
      b) *Neurosyphilis or syphilitic eye disease*: Aqueous crystalline penicillin G 18–24 million units IV for 10–14 days
      c) **If Allergic to Penicillin**
         (1) Allergic patients should be desensitized and treated with penicillin.
         (2) Alternatives to penicillin for primary, secondary, and early latent syphilis include doxycycline 100 mg po 2 times a day for 14 days, Ceftriaxone (Rocephin) 1g IM or IV qd for 8–10 days, or Azithromycin (Zithromax) 2 g po for 1. Late latent syphilis or latent syphilis of unknown duration. Doxycycline 100 mg 2 times a day for 28 days. Neurosyphilis is treated with Ceftriaxone (Rocephin) 2 g IM or IV qd for 10–14 days.

G. **Syphilis in Pregnancy**
   1. Screen all patients for syphilis with RPR at the first prenatal visit. High risk patients should be rescreened at 28–32 weeks and at delivery.
   2. **Treatment**
      a) Penicillin regimens for pregnancy are the same as for nonpregnancy.

b) If the patient is allergic to penicillin, the patient should be desensitized and treated with penicillin in the hospital.

c) The Jarisch-Herxheimer reaction consists of transient fever, chills, arthralgia, headache, and tachycardia because of rapid lysis of spirochetes. 40% of pregnant patients may have transient uterine contractions.

IX. Granuloma Inguinale

A. Diagnosis

1. Granuloma inguinale causes painless, beefy red ulcers. Regional lymphadenopathy is absent.
2. The disease is due to intracellular Klebsiella granulomatis. The organism is difficult to culture.
3. Donovan bodies are visible on biopsy.
4. PCR testing with CLIA verification may be done.

B. Treatment

1. Doxycycline 100 mg 2 times a day ≥3 weeks and until lesions have healed

C. Alternative Regimens

1. Azithromycin (Zithromax) 1 g po weekly for at least 3 weeks or
2. Ciprofloxacin 750 mg, 2 times a day for at least 3 weeks or
3. Erythromycin base 500 mg qid for at least 3 weeks or
4. Trimethoprim-sulfamethoxazole (800 mg/160 mg), 2 times a day for at least 3 weeks and until lesions have healed.

X. Lymphogranuloma Venereum

A. Diagnosis

1. Tender inguinal lymphadenopathy and self-limited genital ulcers. Proctocolitis occurs in homosexuals.
2. LGV is due to Chlamydia trachomatis L1, L2, or L3
3. Laboratory testing: complement fixation titers and C. trachomatis in tissue aspirate.

B. Treatment

1. Doxycycline 100 mg po, 2 times a day for 21 days OR
2. Erythromycin base 500 mg 4 times a day for 21 days

C. Chancroid

1. **Diagnosis**
   a) Chancroid presents with one or more painful genital ulcers;
   b) The patient has no evidence of T. pallidum infection by darkfield examination or serologic testing;
   c) Regional lymphadenopathy
   d) HSV testing of ulcer exudate is negative.
   e) **Definitive diagnosis:**
      (1) Identification of Haemophilus ducreyi on special culture media or
      (2) PCR test

2. **Treatment**
   a) Azithromycin (Zithromax) 1 g po or
   b) Ceftriaxone (Rocephin) 250 mg IM or
   c) Ciprofloxacin 500 mg po 2 times a day for 3 days or
   d) Erythromycin base 500 mg po tid for 7 days.

XI. Pediculosis Pubis (Pubic Lice)

A. Pediculosis presents with pruritus and nits on pubic hair.

B. Recommended Regimens

1. Permethrin 1% cream rinse should be applied to affected areas and washed off after 10 minutes or
2. Pyrethrins with piperonyl butoxide should be applied and washed off after 10 minutes
3. Spinosad (Natroba) apply to pubic hair for 10 minutes, then rinse

4. Sexual partners should be treated.

XII. Scabies

A. Sexually acquired in adults, but sexually acquired not in children. Pruritus is the predominant symptom.

B. **Treatment**
1. Permethrin cream 5% should be applied to all areas of the body from the neck down and washed off after 8–14 hours or
2. Ivermectin 200 μg/kg po and repeat in 2 weeks

Ectopic Pregnancy

Ectopic pregnancy is the most common cause of pregnancy-related maternal death in the first trimester. Ectopic pregnancy occurs in 0.64% of pregnancies.

I. Risk Factors

A. Ectopic pregnancy is associated with tubal damage from pelvic inflammatory disease, previous tubal surgery, prior ectopic pregnancy, and assisted reproductive techniques.

B. Approximately 50% of patients with ectopic pregnancy do not have any risk factors.

II. Contraception and Ectopic Pregnancy

A. All methods of contraception reduce the absolute risk of ectopic pregnancy. Sterilization and intrauterine systems raise the risk of ectopic pregnancy.

III. Sites of Ectopic Pregnancy: Ampullary (70%), isthmic (12%), fimbrial (11.1%), ovarian (3.2%), interstitial or cornual (2.4%), and abdominal (1.3%).

IV. Symptoms of Ectopic Pregnancy

A. Presenting signs include abdominal pain (99%), amenorrhea (74%), and vaginal spotting (56%). Shoulder pain results from diaphragm irritation by hemoperitoneum.

B. Lower abdominal tenderness and rebound tenderness are signs of acute abdomen due to blood in the peritoneum. Surgery is advised regardless of β-hCG level.

C. Hypotension and tachycardia are signs of hemodynamic instability.

V. Differential Diagnosis

A. Causes of vaginal bleeding with a positive pregnancy test include early normal pregnancy and spontaneous abortion.

B. Abortion causes heavy vaginal bleeding and passage of clots or tissue.

VI. Diagnostic Workup

A. A positive urine pregnancy test confirms pregnancy. Gestational weeks should be calculated from the last menstrual period.

B. **Laboratory Studies**
1. **Serum β-hCG**
   a) Normal pregnancy will cause the β-hCG to rise by 53–200% over 2 days and double every 2 days.
   b) If β-hCG ≥1,500–2,000 IU/L (discriminatory zone), a normal intrauterine pregnancy should be visible on vaginal ultrasound.
2. **Other Laboratory Studies**: CBC, type and screen, and metabolic panel.
3. **Vaginal Ultrasound**
   a) Visualization of intrauterine pregnancy excludes ectopic pregnancy. Heterotopic pregnancy is rare unless the pregnancy occurs after assisted reproduction.
   b) Ectopic pregnancy is confirmed if ultrasound demonstrates an extrauterine gestational sac with a yolk sac or embryo.

c) A large volume of fluid in peritoneal cavity suggests a ruptured ectopic pregnancy.

VII. Treatment of Ectopic Pregnancy with Methotrexate

A. Laboratory Studies: CBC, metabolic panel, and serum β-hCG

B. Single dose therapy is less expensive and has fewer side effects. Multi-dose regimen may be used for patients with β-hCG >5,000.

C. **Single-dose Methotrexate Treatment**
   1. Day 1: give methotrexate 50 mg/m^2 IM
   2. Day 4: assess serum β-hCG
   3. Day 7: assess β-hCG. A second dose of methotrexate may be given if the decline in β-hCG is less than 15%
   4. Weekly β-hCG are checked until negative

D. **Favorable Indicators for Methotrexate Therapy**
   1. Absent or mild symptoms
   2. β-hCG less than 5,000
   3. Absent embryonic heart activity
   4. Ectopic gestational mass less than 4 cm

E. **Contraindications to Methotrexate**
   1. Hemodynamic instability with hypotension and tachycardia
   2. Acute bleeding as indicated by a large volume of free fluid in peritoneal cavity
   3. Contraindications to methotrexate include breastfeeding, immunodeficiency, alcoholism, chronic liver disease, renal disease, hematologic or pulmonary disease, peptic ulcer disease, and sensitivity to methotrexate

F. **Side Effects of Methotrexate**
   1. Nausea, vomiting, stomatitis, and conjunctivitis are the most frequent side effects of methotrexate. Bone marrow depression, elevated transaminases, alopecia and pneumonitis are infrequent adverse effects.
   2. Precautions after methotrexate include avoidance of intercourse, vigorous activity, sun exposure, alcohol, folic acid, and NSAIDs. Mild pain is treated with acetaminophen.

G. **Treatment of Abdominal Pain after Methotrexate Therapy**
   1. Pain may be caused by tubal abortion, tubal hematoma, or tubal rupture. Abdominal pain is common 2–3 days after methotrexate.
   2. If the patient has severe abdominal pain, admit the patient for observation. Assess hemoglobin and monitor intraperitoneal fluid with vaginal ultrasound.
   3. Methotrexate failure and tubal rupture requires surgery in 15% of patients.

H. **Surgical Treatment**
   1. **Laparoscopy versus Laparotomy**
      a) Laparoscopy is associated with less blood loss, fewer adhesion, and a shorter hospital stay
      b) Laparotomy is used for hemodynamic instability and hemorrhagic shock.

Spontaneous Abortion

Spontaneous abortion (SAB) is defined as pregnancy loss before 20 weeks' gestation or when the fetus weighs less than 350 grams. Early pregnancy losses occur in one third of pregnancies.

I. Fetal Genetic Abnormalities Associated with Spontaneous Abortion
   A. Genetic abnormalities cause 85% of Spontaneous abortions. Autosomal trisomy is the most frequent abnormal karyotype (50%). The most frequent chromosomal abnormality is 45 X (20%).

II. Maternal Risk Factors for Spontaneous Abortion
   A. Advanced maternal age, prior SAB, irradiation, overweight or underweight, smoking, alcohol and drug abuse, medications, uterine anomalies, cytomegalovirus, parvovirus B19, Toxoplasma, rubella, and Listeria infection

III. Abortion Types and Clinical Features
   A. **Threatened abortion** is uterine bleeding without cervical dilation or effacement. The bleeding is painless.
      1. The pregnancy is likely to continue.
      2. **Inevitable abortion** is uterine bleeding and cervical dilation without expulsion of fetal or placental tissue.
      3. **Incomplete abortion** is an open cervix with partial expulsion of the product of conception
   B. **Complete abortion** is when the product of conception has been completely expelled, the cervix is closed, and bleeding and cramping have ceased.
   C. **Missed abortion** is when the dead fetus remains in the uterus without bleeding or cramping. Consumptive coagulopathy may rarely occur after 5 weeks.
   D. **Septic abortion** is characterized by lower abdominal pain, foul discharge, abdominal tenderness, cervical motion tenderness, fever, and leukocytosis. Septic abortion is treated with immediate evacuation and antibiotics.

IV. Diagnosis
   A. Features of nonviable pregnancy on ultrasound include lack of fetal pole when gestational sac is >2 cm or lack of fetal cardiac activity when the crown rump length is more than 0.5 cm.
   B. A pseudosac is a collection of endometrial secretions, which is frequently asymmetric septated.
   C. Subchorionic hematoma is a risk factor for future placenta abruption and preterm delivery.
   D. Pelvic ultrasound and serum b-hCG may be needed for evaluation of spontaneous abortion.

V. Vaginal Ultrasound Features and b-hCG Levels in Early Pregnancy
   A. 4–5 Weeks: gestational sac (2–5 mm) has a b-hCG of 1,500–3,000
   B. 5–6 Weeks: yolk sac; b-hCG 5,000
   C. 6–7 Weeks: fetal heart activity, crown rump length >5 mm has a b-hCG of 15,000

VI. Treatment of Early Pregnancy Failure
   A. Patients with excessive bleeding, unstable vital signs or infection should be hospitalized. Dilation and curettage should be performed to empty the uterus and stop the bleeding.
   B. The product of conception should be sent to the pathology lab for confirmation.
   C. Give RhD immune globulin (50 mcg up to 12 weeks) if RhD is negative.
   D. The ultrasound should be repeated in 1 week if the POC findings are equivocal.
   E. Expectant management, misoprostol, and dilation and curettage are effective.

VII. Misoprostol (Cytotec)
   A. Misoprostol is safe, effective, and inexpensive. Misoprostol can be given vaginally, orally, or sublingually.
   B. The complete abortion rate 99%.

C. Side effects of misoprostol include diarrhea, nausea, vomiting, and fever.

D. **Vaginal Misoprostol**
   1. 800 µg into posterior fornix. Follow-up visit in 2–5 days, give second dose if abortion incomplete. Vacuum aspiration is done if still incomplete on day 8.
   2. 71% success rate with 1 dose and 84% with 2 doses by day 8.

E. **Oral and Sublingual Misoprostol**
   1. 600 µg PO. Follow-up at 48h and 1 week. Success rate is 96% in incomplete abortion
   2. 400 µg PO and repeat in 3h with a total dose 800 µg, follow-up at 48h. If unsuccessful after 48 hours, give another 800 µg PO; 73.6% success rate for missed abortion.
   3. 600 µg sublingually q3h for a maximum of 3 doses with a success rate of 87.5%.

VIII. **Dilation and Curettage**
   A. Dilation and curettage is an effective treatment for early pregnancy failure.
   B. Dilation and Curettage may rarely be complicated by uterine perforation and infection, cervical laceration, and anesthesia complications.

IX. **Follow-up**
   A. Serum β-hCG usually becomes negative 2–4 weeks after complete abortion. Follow the urine pregnancy test to negative or follow the serum b-hCG to nondetectable.
   B. The patient should wait 2–3 months before attempting to conceive again.

X. **Recurrent Abortions**
   A. Recurrent abortion is defined as 2–3 or more consecutive miscarriages.
   B. After 3 losses, an evaluation is advised.
   C. **Evaluation of Recurrent Abortions**
      1. Systemic evaluation includes thyroid disorder, diabetes mellitus, and polycystic ovarian syndrome.
      2. Anatomic uterine abnormalities are assessed with pelvic ultrasound, sonohysterogram, hysterosalpingogram, or hysteroscopy
      3. Coagulation evaluation is with anticardiolipin IgG and IgM, lupus anticoagulant.
      4. Karyotype study of the product of conception should assess for chromosomal anomaly. Both partners should be assessed for balanced translocation or inversion.
   D. **Management of Recurrent Abortions**
      1. The probability of a successful next pregnancy is 70%.
      2. Prophylactic heparin and low dose aspirin may be used for pregnancies with antiphospholipid syndrome.

Acute Pelvic Pain

I. **Evaluation of Acute Pelvic Pain**
   A. Perform a history assessment for pelvic pain, fever, nausea, vomiting, constipation, and dysuria.
   B. **Abdominal and Pelvic Examination**
      1. Assess for abdominal distension, focal tenderness, rebound tenderness, and pelvic masses.
      2. Cervical motion tenderness indicates infection, hemoperitoneum, or inflammation.
      3. Purulent discharge from cervical os is a sign of pelvic inflammatory disease.

II. **Pregnancy Test.** Urine pregnancy test will classify the disorder as pregnancy-related or related-related.

III. **Imaging**
   A. Pelvic ultrasound is the imaging for pelvic conditions.
   B. Moderate or large volume of free fluid indicates acute hemorrhage and the need for surgery.
   C. CT with contrast is better than ultrasound for non-gynecologic conditions, such as appendicitis and diverticulitis.

IV. **Differential Diagnosis**
   A. Gynecological disorders include pelvic inflammatory disease, ectopic pregnancy, abortion, adnexal torsion, ruptured ovarian cyst, endometriosis, and degenerating fibroids.
   B. Non-gynecologic disorders include appendicitis, cystitis, urolithiasis, diverticulitis, ulcerative colitis, and irritable bowel syndrome.

V. **Pelvic Inflammatory Disease**
   A. **Etiology and Epidemiology**
      1. PID is an acute infection of the upper genital tract, including endometritis, salpingitis, tuboovarian abscess, and pelvic peritonitis.
      2. Pelvic inflammatory disease is a polymicrobial infection caused by bacteria from the vagina and cervix. The initiating microorganisms are usually C. trachomatis and N. gonorrhoeae.
      3. Sexually active women 15–25 years of age are at highest risk. Other risk factors include multiple partners, young age at first intercourse, and prior pelvic inflammatory disease.
   B. **Clinical Manifestation and Diagnosis**
      1. PID presents with acute lower abdominal pain, vaginal bleeding or discharge, fever, nausea, and vomiting.
      2. Exam demonstrates bilateral lower abdominal tenderness. Rebound tenderness suggests peritonitis. Cervical motion tenderness and adnexal tenderness are common findings.
      3. Fitz-Hugh-Curtis syndrome is right upper quadrant pain and tenderness due to perihepatic infection from PID. Liver enzymes can be mildly elevated.
      4. Ultrasound differentiates tubo-ovarian abscess from adnexal mass.
      5. Laparoscopy can confirm pelvic inflammatory disease if other surgical conditions, appendicitis or ovarian torsion, cannot be excluded.
   C. **Treatment of Pelvic Inflammatory Disease**
      1. **Criteria for Hospitalization**
         a) Appendicitis cannot be excluded;
         b) Patient is pregnant;
         c) Patient has severe illness, nausea and vomiting, or high fever.
         d) Tubo-ovarian abscess
      2. **Parenteral Treatment**
      3. **Regimen A**
         a) Cefotetan 2g IV q12h or cefoxitin 2g IV q6h PLUS
         b) Doxycycline 100 mg po or IV q12h
      4. **Regimen B**
         a) Clindamycin 900 mg IV q8h PLUS
         b) Gentamicin 2 mg/kg IV or IM, followed by 3–5 mg/kg q24h.
      5. **Alternative Parenteral Regimens**
         a) Ampicillin/sulbactam 3g IV q6h PLUS doxycycline 100 mg po or IV q12h
         b) Continue IV antibiotics 24 hours after improvement.
      6. **Oral Treatment**
         a) Ceftriaxone (Rocephin) 250 mg IM and doxycycline 100 mg po 2 times a day for 14 days with Metronidazole (Flagyl) 500 mg po 2 times a day for 14 days.

       b) Cefoxitin 2g IM and probenecid 1 g po and doxycycline 100 mg po 2 times a day for 14 days with Metronidazole (Flagyl) 500 mg po 2 times a day for 14 days.

       c) Ceftizoxime or cefotaxime PLUS doxycycline 100 mg po 2 times a day for 14 days with Metronidazole (Flagyl) 500 mg po 2 times a day for 14 days.

7. **Alternative Oral Regimen**

       a) Ceftriaxone (Rocephin) 250 mg IM and Azithromycin (Zithromax) 1 g po weekly for 2 doses and Metronidazole (Flagyl) 500 mg 2 times a day for 14 days.

       b) Amoxicillin/clavulanic acid plus doxycycline and Metronidazole (Flagyl) for anaerobic coverage.

       c) Fluoroquinolones are not advised because of drug-resistant gonorrhea. May be considered if parenteral cephalosporin is not feasible. Complete a culture for gonorrhea after therapy. Levofloxacin 500 mg po qd or ofloxacin 400 mg po 2 times a day for 14 d with Metronidazole (Flagyl) 500 mg po 2 times a day for 14 days. Also add Azithromycin (Zithromax) 2 g.

D. **Treatment of Tubo-ovarian Abscess**

    1. Antibiotic regimen for severe pelvic inflammatory disease or tuboovarian abscess:

       a) Clindamycin 900 mg IV every 8 hours and Ceftriaxone (Rocephin) 1 gram IV q12h or clindamycin and aminoglycoside and ampicillin

       b) Oral antibiotics at discharge: amoxicillin/clavulanate 875 mg 2 times a day or trimethoprim/ sulfamethoxazole 160/800 mg 2 times a day and Metronidazole (Flagyl) 500 mg 2 times a day for 14 days.

    2. Consider drainage if not responding to antibiotics or abscess >10 cm. Transvaginal drainage is performed under ultrasound guidance.

    3. Sex partners should be treated.

VI. Ovarian Torsion

A. Ovarian torsion presents with sudden and severe, lower abdominal pain, nausea, vomiting, severe adrenal tenderness, and rebound tenderness.

B. Pelvic ultrasound demonstrates an enlarged ovary. Ovarian cysts and tumors can be present. Malignancy is rare in children and young women.

C. Doppler demonstrates reduced or absent venous flow. Arterial flow can be compromised. Normal flow does not exclude torsion.

D. **Treatment**

    1. Laparoscopy confirms the diagnosis. Clinical findings are nonspecific.

    2. Surgical management is detorsion. The ovary is usually functional and should be left in-situ.

    3. Oophorectomy may be completed if ovary is grossly necrotic or if a tumor is present.

VII. Ruptured Ovarian Cysts

A. Corpus luteum cyst rupture is common and causes mild lower abdominal pain, lasting a few hours or a day.

B. Ruptured corpus luteum cyst usually occurs in the luteal phase.

C. Lower abdominal tenderness and rebound tenderness are common. Cervical motion tenderness can sometimes be present.

D. **Ultrasound:** An ovarian cyst and pelvic free fluid suggests hemorrhage.

E. Treatment of ovarian cyst is analgesia. Laparoscopy may be indicated if ovarian torsion cannot be excluded.

Chronic Pelvic Pain

I. **Clinical Evaluation**
  A. Chronic pelvic pain affects 15% of women.
  B. **Gynecologic Causes of Chronic Pelvic Pain**
    1. Endometriosis, pelvic inflammatory disease, cancer, adhesion, leiomyoma, adenomyosis, dysmenorrhea, ovulatory pain, adnexal cysts, chronic ectopic pregnancy, endometrial or cervical polyps, and chronic endometritis
  C. **Non-gynecologic Causes of Chronic Pelvic Pain**
    1. Urologic: painful bladder syndrome, cancer, urethral syndrome, uninhibited bladder contraction, urethral diverticulum, urinary tract infection, and urolithiasis.
    2. GI: Constipation, cancer, IBD, irritable bowel syndrome, colitis, bowel obstruction, and diverticular disease
    3. Musculoskeletal: Fibromyalgia and myofascial pain.
    4. Mental: Depression, somatization
II. **Evaluation of Chronic Pelvic Pain**
  A. History and physical exam including rectal exam
  B. Pregnancy test, CBC, urinalysis and culture, and pelvic ultrasound
  C. Laparoscopy if indicated
III. **Painful Bladder Syndrome**
  A. Painful bladder syndrome was previously called interstitial cystitis.
  B. Possible etiology is that defects of glycosaminoglycan layer lead to altered uroepithelial permeability and allow irritants to enter the bladder wall.
IV. **Diagnosis**
  A. Suprapubic pain occurs with bladder filling, resulting in frequent urination, nocturia, and urgency.
  B. Physical findings include tenderness in suprapubic area and anterior vaginal wall.
  C. Differential Diagnosis: urinary tract infection, irritable bowel syndrome, overactive bladder, and endometriosis
  D. Laboratory Evaluation: urinalysis and culture, post-void residual, cystoscopy for patients with hematuria
V. **Cystoscopy, Hydrodistension, and Bladder Biopsy**
  A. Cystoscopy is not routinely needed for diagnosis of PBS because of a 60% underdiagnosis rate of cystoscopy.
  B. Hydrodistention involves filling the bladder with normal saline to a pressure of 70 cm of water under anesthesia. Symptom relief for 3–6 months in 90% of patients.
VI. **Treatment**
  A. **Bladder Retraining** gradually increase voiding intervals to increase bladder capacity. Avoid food or drinks.
  B. **Medications**
    1. Pentosan polysulfate sodium (Elmiron) 100 mg po tid or 200 mg 2 times a day; 6–8 months of treatment with 65–70% response rate. Reversible alopecia occurs in 4%.
    2. Amitriptyline 25 mg po qhs and increase up to 100 mg qhs. Hydroxyzine 25 mg po qhs, up to 100 mg qhs
  C. **Intravesical Therapy**
    1. Heparin 40,000 units or Elmiron 100 mg, 8 ml of 2% lidocaine, and 3 ml of 8.4% $NaHCO_3$. Fluid remains in bladder for 15–30 min. 2–3 treatments a week for 2–3 weeks has a success rate of 80%.
    2. Other agents: dimethyl sulfoxide (DMSO), BCG, and hyaluronic acid

Menstrual Disorders

I. Primary Dysmenorrhea
  A. Painful menses in the absence of pathology.
  B. Primary dysmenorrhea is common in the first 3 years after menarche and improves after a full-term pregnancy.

II. Treatment
  A. Start NSAID at the onset of menstruation and continue for 2–3 days.
   1. Naproxen 500 mg po 2 times a day
   2. Ibuprofen 400 mg po q6–8h
   3. Ketoprofen 50 mg po q6–8h
   4. Mefenamic acid 500 mg po for 1 then 250 mg q6h
  B. Oral contraceptive if contraception is desired

III. Premenstrual Disorder
  A. **Common Premenstrual Complaints**
   1. Irritability, mood swings, depression, anxiety, and low self-esteem
   2. Physical and behavioral: bloating, breast tenderness, headaches, hot flashes, insomnia, fatigue, appetite change, decreased interests in usual activities, and poor concentration.
  B. **Diagnosis**
  C. **Premenstrual Dysphoric Disorder**
   1. At least five of the following symptoms are present a week before menses and remit a few days after the onset of menses. **Core symptoms:** depressed mood or dysphoria, anxiety or tension, affective lability, and irritability. **Others:** marked lack of energy, hypersomnia or insomnia, feeling overwhelmed, reduced interest in usual activities, concentration difficulties, other physical symptoms (e.g., breast tenderness, bloating, headache, muscle pain)
   2. Symptoms must interfere with work, school, usual activities, or relationships.

IV. Premenstrual Syndrome
  A. Premenstrual symptoms do not meet criteria for premenstrual dysphoric disorder.
  B. PMS is associated with more than one of the following symptoms during the 5 days before menses in each of the three prior menstrual cycles with resolution within 4 days of the onset of menses: Depression, angry outbursts, irritability, anxiety, confusion, social withdrawal, breast tenderness, abdominal bloating, headache, change in appetite, and swollen ankles.

V. Treatment of Premenstrual Symptoms
  A. Calcium, diet change, and exercise
  B. Selective serotonin-reuptake inhibitors.
  C. Anxiolytics: Alprazolam IR 0.25 to 0.5 mg tid or alprazolam ER 0.5 mg qd. Buspirone 5 mg 2 times a day.
  D. Oral contraceptive: Beyaz (drospirenone 3 mg/ethinyl estradiol 20 mcg/levomefolate calcium 451 mcg for 24 days and levomefolate calcium 451 mcg for 4 days) is approved for premenstrual dysphoric disorder.

Endometriosis

I. **Epidemiology**
  A. Endometriosis is the presence of endometrial tissue outside the uterus. The most frequent location is the pelvic peritoneum, 10% of cases may involve urinary or GI tract.
  B. Endometriosis affects 6–10% women of reproductive age with an average age of diagnosis of 28 years.

II. **Clinical Presentation**
  A. Chronic pelvic pain can be minimal to debilitating with dysmenorrhea and dyspareunia, dysuria or dyschezia.
  B. Dysmenorrhea begins before and persists through the menses. Dyspareunia suggests immobility of the uterus or involvement of the cul-de-sac.
  C. Severe endometriosis is associated with infertility.
  D. **Pelvic Examination**
    1. Non-specific findings on pelvic examination include reduced uterine mobility and retroverted uterus. Nodules on the uterosacral ligament or rectovaginal septum are infrequent.
    2. Endometrioma may form an adnexal mass.
  E. **Imaging.** Pelvic ultrasound is the preferred imaging, but ultrasound is nonspecific. Endometrioma appear as a cyst containing homogeneous echo and a ground glass-appearance.
  F. **Laboratory Studies.** CA 125 may be elevated, but CA125 lacks sensitivity and specificity.
  G. **Laparoscopy**
    1. Laparoscopy is the gold standard for diagnosis of endometriosis
    2. Three types of endometriosis include (1) superficial peritoneal implants (brown, bluish or red nodules on the pelvic peritoneum and ovaries), (2) endometrioma, and (3) deep infiltrating endometriosis.
    3. Biopsy is not required for the diagnosis.

III. **Medical Treatment**
  A. Medical treatment reduces pelvic pain, but medical treatment does not improve infertility.
  B. **NSAIDs:** Naproxen, ibuprofen, and mefenamic acid.
  C. **Combined oral contraceptives**
    1. Cyclic and continuous regimens can be used.
    2. Continuous regimens use monophasic pills for 6–12 months (without placebo pills). Breakthrough bleeding is treated with conjugated estrogen, 1.25 mg qd for one week or estradiol 2.0 mg qd for 1 week.
  D. **Progestins**
    1. Progestins provide similar pain relief as GnRH agonists.
    2. Norethindrone acetate 5 or 10 mg po qd
    3. Medroxyprogesterone acetate (Provera) 20–100 mg po qd
    4. Megestrol 20–40 mg po qd
    5. Depo-Provera 150 mg IM every 3 months. Or Depo-SubQ Provera 104
    6. Etonogestrel releasing implant
    7. Levonorgestrel intrauterine system (Mirena) is as effective as GnRH analogues
  E. **GnRH Agonists**
    1. Leuprolide acetate (Depo-Lupron) 11.25 mg IM every 3 months or 3.75 mg IM every month
    2. Nafarelin intranasal spray 400 to 600 µg daily

3. **Side Effects**
   a) Menopausal symptoms, such as hot flashes and vaginal dryness, because of hypoestrogenism.
   b) Decreased bone density develops after more than 6-months of treatment.
   c) GnRH treatment should be limited to 6–12 months due to side effects.
4. **Add-back Regimen**
   a) Add-back regimen minimizes hypoestrogenic side effects.
   b) Norethindrone acetate 5 mg (Aygestin) po qd is the most frequently used regimen.
F. **Aromatase Inhibitor**: Premenopausal: letrozole 2.5 mg or anastrozole 1 mg po qd. An oral contraceptive, progestin, such as norethindrone acetate 2.5 mg qd, or GnRH agonist should be added for ovarian suppression.
G. **Surgical Treatment**
   1. Excision and ablation may not be effective for mild endometriosis. Excision and ablation have similar outcomes in early diseases.
   2. Surgery may not improve infertility in severe endometriosis because surgery can increase scar formation. Resection of endometrioma can diminish ovarian reserves.
   3. Hysterectomy with bilateral salpingo-oophorectomy is used for women who no longer desire fertility. Hormone replacement therapy is an option after hysterectomy and bilateral salpingo-oophorectomy.

Uterine Leiomyoma

Uterine leiomyoma are presents in 20-25% of reproductive age women. The prevalence of uterine Leiomyoma is 2–3 times higher in African American than White women. Uterine leiomyoma usually regresses after menopause.

I. **Diagnosis**
   A. Uterine leiomyomas (fibroids) are most commonly asymptomatic (70%) and found during pelvic exam.
   B. Large fibroids may cause menorrhagia, pelvic pressure or pain, bladder dysfunctions, and infertility.
   C. Submucosal fibroids cause significant uterine bleeding.
   D. Vaginal ultrasound is used to evaluate fibroids, uterus, and adnexa.
II. **Treatment**
   A. Asymptomatic or symptomatic patients nearing menopause are observed.
   B. Treatment is indicated for abnormal uterine bleeding, anemia, pelvic pain or pressure, infertility associated with cavity distortion, and possible malignancy
III. **Medical Therapy**
   A. GnRH agonist are used preoperatively for large uterine leiomyoma and anemia. Leuprolide (Lupron) for 2–3 months increases hemoglobin and hematocrit, decreases uterine size, and decreases surgical blood loss.
   B. Mifepristone decreases fibroid size, uterine bleeding, and dysmenorrhea. 5 mg po qd for 6 months reduced uterine size by 47%.
   C. Levonorgestrel intrauterine system (Mirena) is an option for heavy menses if the cavity is normal in shape.
   D. NSAIDs relieve pain and bleeding.

IV. Surgical Treatment
  A. **Hysterectomy** is a definitive therapy.
  B. **Myomectomy** is used for women who want to retain their uterus. Myomectomy has a 50% recurrence rate in 5 years. The risk of uterine rupture prior to labor after abdominal myomectomy is very low. Cesarean is recommended if the uterine cavity was entered during surgery.
  C. **Hysteroscopy** is used for removal of submucosal leiomyomas.
  D. **Uterine Artery Embolization**
    1. Uterine leiomyoma may be treated with bilateral embolization with polyvinyl alcohol, Gelfoam, or Embosphere microspheres
    2. Uterine artery embolization decreases menstrual flow and decreases symptoms related to a large uterus. The overall failure rate is 9.3%.
    3. Uterine artery embolization is contraindicated in women desiring fertility.
  E. **Thermoablation with MRI-Guided Ultrasound (ExAblate)** is less invasive than uterine artery embolization and may shrink the fibroids by 20%.
  F. **Uterine Leiomyomas and Infertility**
    1. Submucosal fibroids and intramural fibroids may impair implantation of the zygote.
    2. Myomectomy may cause postoperative intrauterine adhesions and weaken the uterine wall.
V. Adenomyosis
  A. Adenomyosis is the growth of endometrial glands and stroma inside myometrium.
  B. 50% of patients are asymptomatic. 50% have dysmenorrhea, menorrhagia, and dyspareunia. Adenomyosis occurs between 35 to 50 years age.
  C. Pelvic exam demonstrates a diffusely enlarged uterus (2–3 times normal).
  D. Diagnosis: Ultrasound will demonstrate fibroids. Diagnosis requires histology.
  E. Treatment: may try oral contraceptives or LNG-intrauterine system for menorrhagia. The definitive treatment of myomas is hysterectomy.

Adnexal Mass

Adnexal masses are the most commonly found incidentally on ultrasound or CT. The vast majority of adnexal masses are benign in women of reproductive age.

I. Benign Adnexal Cysts
  A. The most frequent adnexal cyst is the follicular cyst. Ultrasound demonstrates a simple, translucent, and thin-walled cyst in the ovarian cortex. A normal follicle (up to 2.5 cm) is normal.
  B. Corpus luteum cysts are less common and have a complex ultrasound appearance. Ruptured hemorrhagic cysts can cause acute pelvic pain.
II. Benign Adnexal Tumors include teratoma, serous cystadenoma, mucinous cystadenoma, fibroma, and cystic mesothelioma
III. Infections include hydrosalpinx or tubal ovarian abscess, and appendiceal abscess
IV. Ovarian Malignancies include epithelial ovarian cancer, borderline or low malignant potential tumor, germ cell and sex-cord stromal tumors, and metastatic cancer.
V. Non-gynecologic Masses include pelvic kidney, retroperitoneal tumors, and colon cancer

VI. Evaluation of Adnexal of Masses
  A. Adnexal masses are imaged with pelvic ultrasound. CT can detect cancer metastasis if malignancy is suspected.
  B. **Characteristics Suggesting Malignancy**
    1. Ascites and omental caking
    2. Bilateral masses
    3. Complex mass with solid components or excrescences
    4. Nodular or fixed mass
    5. Pelvic masses in premenarchal girls and postmenopausal women
  C. **CA 125 and Other Tumor Markers**
    1. CA 125
      a) CA 125 is a glycoprotein, which is elevated in more than 80% of nonmucinous epithelial ovarian cancers. CA 125 is also elevated in breast, endometrial, lung, and pancreatic cancers, endometriosis, cirrhosis, and pelvic inflammatory disease, and pregnancy.
      b) CA 125 is a useful marker for ovarian cancer follow-up
    2. CEA and CA 19-9 are elevated in mucinous ovarian cancers
    3. AFP, hCG, and LDH are sometimes elevated in malignant germ cell tumors
    4. Inhibin A and B are elevated in granulosa cell tumor.

VII. Treatment of Ovarian Cysts
  A. **Premenopausal Women**
    1. Ovarian cysts are usually related to ovulation.
    2. The patient with an ovarian cyst should be observed for 8 weeks if the cyst is <10 cm, mobile, and unilateral. The ultrasound should be repeated in 2 months.
  B. **Indications for Surgery for an Ovarian Cyst**
    1. Cyst size >10 cm
    2. Solid ovarian mass, or papillary vegetation in the cyst wall
    3. Ascites
    4. Suspected torsion or rupture
  C. **Surgical Approach**: Laparoscopy is the preferred surgical approach for ovarian cysts.
  D. **Postmenopausal Women**
  E. **Simple Adnexal Cyst**
    1. Unilocular and less than 10 cm
    2. No ovarian malignancy
    3. Monitor pelvic exam, ultrasound, and CA 125 every 3 months until resolution. Spontaneous resolution occurs in about 70% in 3 months. Surgery is indicated if the cyst persists.
  F. **Complex Adnexal Cysts** are managed surgically with cystectomy.
  G. **Adnexal Mass in Pregnancy**
    1. During pregnancy, most adnexal masses are physiological cysts, teratomas, and paratubal cysts. Hyperreactio luteinalis and leuteoma only occur in pregnancy and resolve spontaneously after delivery.
    2. Cysts usually resolve spontaneously during pregnancy. Expectant management is advised for incidental adnexal masses. Laparoscopy is performed to assess ovarian torsion or malignancy.
  H. **Ovarian Teratoma**
    1. Ovarian teratoma is the most common ovarian tumor in women of 20–40 years of age; 10% of teratomas are bilateral.
    2. Teratomas are classified into mature, immature, or highly specialized. Malignant immature teratoma accounts for 1% of teratomas.
    3. Benign cystic teratoma is also called dermoid cyst. The benign cystic teratoma contains hair, sebaceous material, neural tissue, teeth, cartilage, bone and adipose tissue, thyroid gland, and epithelium.

4. Struma ovarii is a rare teratoma, containing predominant thyroid tissue. Less than 5% of struma ovarii cause thyrotoxicosis. Carcinoid teratoma is rare and may cause flushing, diarrhea, abdominal cramping, and cardiac disease.

Polycystic Ovarian Syndrome

Polycystic ovarian syndrome affects 5% of women of reproductive age and is a common cause of infertility.

I. **Diagnostic Criteria for Polycystic Ovarian Syndrome**
   A. Menstrual irregularity including anovulation or oligomenorrhea AND
   B. Clinical and/or biochemical signs of hyperandrogenism (hirsutism, acne, or elevated serum androgens), and exclusion of other etiologies (congenital adrenal hyperplasia, androgen-secreting tumor, Cushing's, and elevated prolactin)
II. **Evaluation**
   A. Anovulation and polycystic ovaries are associated with obesity, metabolic syndrome, insulin resistance, hyperinsulinemia, hyperandrogenism, dyslipidemia, hirsutism, acne, increased risks of endometrial and breast cancer, diabetes, and cardiovascular disease.
   B. Laboratory testing: Hemoglobin A1c, lipid profile, TSH, and prolactin.
   C. Endometrial biopsy if chronic anovulation has been present.
III. **Treatment of Polycystic Ovarian Syndrome**
   A. **Lifestyle Modification**
      1. Weight loss reduces blood insulin and androgen level, restores ovulation and menses, and improves abnormal vaginal bleeding, infertility, and hirsutism.
      2. Reduce diet to 500–1000 kcal/day. Increase consumption of whole-grain breads and cereals, and increase fruits and vegetables
      3. Exercise for more than 30 minutes per day.
   B. **Menstrual Regulation**
      1. Oral contraceptives, contraceptive patch, vaginal ring, or progesterone intrauterine system if contraception is needed.
      2. Endometrial protection is indicated if contraception is not desired: Provera 10 mg for 10–14 days a month or micronized progesterone (Prometrium) 200 mg qhs for 10–12 days a month.
   C. **Metformin**
      1. Frequently used to improve glucose tolerance and ovulation in women with insulin resistance.
      2. Dosage: 850 mg PO 2 times a day.
   D. **Statins**
      1. Statins reduce total cholesterol and LDL.
      2. Simvastatin, 20 mg once a day is more effective than metformin in lowering testosterone and DHEAS.

Abnormal Uterine Bleeding

Abnormal uterine bleeding is the most frequent gynecological complaint.

I. **Normal and Abnormal Menstrual Cycles**
   A. Normal cycle length: 21–35 days
   B. Average duration of menses is 4–5 days (>7 days is abnormal)
   C. Normal blood loss per cycle is 35 ml (abnormal is >80 ml)

II. Terminology of Abnormal Menstrual Cycles

A. **Menorrhagia** is heavy menstrual bleeding of more than 80 mL. Increased flow or duration with normal intervals.

B. **Metrorrhagia** is intermenstrual or irregular intervals of bleeding.

C. **Menometrorrhagia** is increased flow or duration of flow with irregular intervals.

D. **Oligomenorrhea** is menstrual intervals of more than 35 days.

E. **Polymenorrhea** is menstrual intervals of less than 21 days.

III. Differential Diagnosis of Abnormal Uterine Bleeding

A. **Structural Etiologies Associated with ovulatory bleeding (menorrhagia) and intermenstrual spotting**

1. Polyps (endometrial or cervical polyp) may present with prolonged and excessive regular bleeding in an ovulatory woman. Polyps are also a common cause of postmenopausal bleeding. Polyps are often asymptomatic, and spontaneous regression may occur if less than 10 mm. Endometrial polyps are suggested by pelvic ultrasound and confirmed by sonohysterogram or hysteroscopy.

2. Adenomyosis may cause abnormal uterine bleeding.

3. Leiomyoma: submucosal leiomyoma cause abnormal uterine bleeding.

4. Malignancy and hyperplasia: cervical cancer and endometrial cancer or hyperplasia may cause uterine bleeding.

B. **Non-structural Etiologies**

1. Coagulopathy: von Willebrand disease, platelet disorder, and leukemia may cause uterine bleeding.

2. Ovulatory dysfunction associated with adolescence, perimenopause, obesity, polycystic ovarian syndrome, and hypothyroidism may cause uterine bleeding

3. Endometrial: inflammation, infection and vascular abnormalities may cause abnormal uterine bleeding

4. Iatrogenic causes of AUB include medications and medical devices

IV. Age-Based Differential Diagnosis of Abnormal Uterine Bleeding

A. Age 13—18: causes of AUB include anovulation, hormonal contraceptives, pregnancy, pelvic infection, coagulopathy, or tumors

B. Age 19—39: pregnancy, leiomyomas or polyps, anovulation, contraception, or endometrial hyperplasia.

C. Age 40 to menopause: anovulation, leiomyomas or polyps, hyperplasia or endometrial cancer

V. Evaluation

A. History, physical exam, and pelvic exam

B. Cyclic (ovulatory) or noncyclic (anovulatory): Regular periods with premenstrual symptoms indicate ovulation. Heavy bleeding in ovulating women may be related to intrauterine pathology. Anovulatory bleeding occurs every few months and is irregular, heavy and prolonged. Postcoital bleeding may result from cervicitis, ectropion, cervical polyp or cervical cancer

C. **Laboratory Studies**: Pregnancy test, CBC, and TSH. Pap smear, Chlamydia, PTT, and fibrinogen

D. **Endometrial Biopsy**

1. Endometrial biopsy is usually completed to exclude endometrial hyperplasia and cancer. Endometrial biopsy on cycle day 18 or later can assess if ovulation occurred. A secretory endometrium confirms that ovulation has occurred.

2. Endometrial biopsy is the first test for women older than 45 years. Endometrial biopsy should be done in patients less than 45 if the woman has had prolonged exposure to unopposed estrogen, such as with obesity or polycystic ovarian syndrome, and anovulation.

E. **Pelvic Ultrasound**
   1. Ultrasound is indicated when anatomic etiologies are suspected.
   2. An endometrial stripe ≤5 mm indicates that malignancy is unlikely. Endometrial thickness is of limited value in premenopausal women.
   3. Saline infusion sonohysterography is useful for diagnosis of intrauterine polyps or fibroids.

F. **Heavy Menstrual Bleeding in Adolescents**
   1. Heavy menstrual bleeding in adolescents is usually because of anovulatory cycles
   2. Initial laboratory evaluation: CBC, INR, aPTT, and fibrinogen for clotting factor deficiency
   3. If von Willebrand disease is suspected, check VWF ristocetin cofactor assay, VWF antigen, and factor VIII activity.

VI. Medical Treatment of Anovulatory Bleeding

A. **For Females Desiring Contraception**
   1. Oral contraceptives are the first-line therapy
   2. Depo-provera 150 mg IM every 3 months is an option
   3. Levonorgestrel intrauterine device is the most effective treatment of menorrhagia.

B. **For Women Not Desiring Contraception**
   1. NSAIDs should be started at the onset of menses and continue through the menses. Bleeding usually decreases by 40%. Naproxen 500 mg 2 times a day. Ibuprofen 600 mg every 6–12 hours. Mefenamic acid 250–500 mg every 6–12 hours.
   2. **Tranexamic Acid (Lysteda)**
      a) Tranexamic acid is an oral antifibrinolytic agent for menorrhagia, which reduces menstrual bleeding by one-third.
      b) Dosage is two 650 mg tabs three times daily (3,900 mg/day) for 5 days when the period starts.
      c) Side effects include menstrual cramps, headache or back pain.
      d) Provera 10 mg qd or Prometrium 200 mg qhs for 10–15 days each month for Endometrial Protection.

C. **Acute Moderate or Severe Bleeding**
   1. Admit if hemoglobin is <8 mg/dL or hemodynamically unstable. Blood transfusion may be needed if symptomatic.
   2. Estrogen or estrogen combined with progestin promotes hemostasis by inducing endometrial proliferation. Use progestin-only method when estrogen is contraindicated.

D. **Combined Oral Contraceptives:** Oral contraceptive 3 times a day should be taken for 1 week then once a day for 3 weeks.

E. **Estrogen Therapy**
   1. **Intravenous Estrogen**
      a) Conjugated estrogens 25 mg IV q4–6hr. Bleeding subsides within 24h. Then start conjugated estrogen 2.5 mg po q6h for 21–26 days. Add provera 10 mg once a day for the last 10 days.
      b) Initiate long-term management with oral contraceptive or progestins.
   2. Oral Estrogen
      a) Conjugated estrogen 2.5 mg or estradiol 2 mg q4–6h until bleeding subsides. Taper to once a day for 7 days after bleeding stops. Then start an oral contraceptive daily.

F. **Surgery**
   1. **Dilation and Curettage**
      a) Rapidly controls profuse uterine bleeding in hemodynamically unstable patients.
      b) D&C may result in incomplete removal of an intrauterine lesion. Medical therapy is often needed after dilation and curettage.

c) **Hysteroscopy and Endometrial Ablation**
d) Hysteroscopy provides definitive diagnosis and treatment of intra-uterine pathology.
e) Preparations: Give misoprostol 200-400 mcg po or vaginally the night before surgery to facilitate cervical dilation. Hysteroscopy should be scheduled during the follicular phase.

2. **Indications**
   a) Chronic menorrhagia
   b) Acute uterine bleeding and failed medical therapy

3. **Contraindications**
   a) Endometrial hyperplasia or cancer
   b) Desires future fertility
   c) Pregnancy
   d) Acute pelvic inflammatory disease

4. **Relative Contraindications**
   a) Postmenopausal bleeding
   b) Abnormal bleeding because of tamoxifen
   c) Uterine size more than 12 weeks
   d) Submucosal fibroids larger than 3 cm

5. **Preoperative Evaluation and Consent**
   a) The procedure reduces menstrual flow, but may not achieve amenorrhea. Amenorrhea rate is 14% to 55%.
   b) Endometrial ablation is not a contraceptive measure. Contraception is required if patient does not have bilateral tubal ligation.
   c) Laparoscopic bilateral tubal ligation can be completed with endometrial ablation.
   d) Pretreatment with GnRH (Lupron 3.75 mg IM per month for 1–2 months) is advised for all the endometrial ablation devices except NovaSure.

6. **Hysterectomy** is the definitive treatment for heavy uterine bleeding. Indicated if other therapies fail.

Hirsutism

I. Definitions
A. Hirsutism is defined as excessive growth of male-pattern facial and body hair. Hirsutism without hyperandrogenemia is known as idiopathic hirsutism.
B. Virilization includes clitoromegaly, deep voice, balding, and hypermuscularity. Virilization is associated with rare androgen-producing tumors.

II. Initial Workup
A. Indications for Androgen Testing
1. Moderate or severe hirsutism
2. Sudden onset or rapidly progressive hirsutism
3. Hirsutism with irregular menses or infertility, virilization, central obesity, or acanthosis nigricans

B. Initial Testing
1. Pelvic ultrasound
2. Prolactin and TSH
3. Dehydroepiandrosterone sulfate (DHEAS): normal level rules out adrenal disease. DHEAS is slightly elevated in polycystic ovarian syndrome. ADHEAS level of >700 µg/dl indicates an androgen-producing tumor.
4. Early morning 17alpha-hydroxyprogesterone. Congenital adrenal hyperplasia due to 21-hydroxylase deficiency is present if 17. Alpha-

hydroprogesterone is more than 800 ng/dL. Perform a ACTH stimulation test if 17-OHP is more than 200 ng/dL.
5. Screen for Cushing syndrome with a 24-hr urinary free cortisol.

III. Testing for Hyperandrogenemia
A. Androgen-producing tumor is indicated by an early morning plasma testosterone >150 ng/dl.
B. Free testosterone level >6.85 pg/ml and/or an 11 desoxycotisol >7 ng/ml are the most sensitive and specific tests for an androgen secreting adrenal tumor

IV. Treatment of Hirsutism
A. **Combined oral contraceptives**
   1. Initial therapy is an oral contraceptive for 6 months. Add antiandrogen therapy if an oral contraceptive is not effective.
   2. Oral contraceptive decreases luteinizing hormone and raises sex hormone-binding globulin and reduces testosterone production and reduces free testosterone.
B. Avoid oral contraceptives with a high androgenic progestin.
C. **Antiandrogen Therapy**
   1. **Spironolactone**
      a) Spironolactone inhibits ovarian and adrenal androgen production and blocks the androgen receptors in hair follicles. Spironolactone decreases DHT by inhibiting 5 alpha-reductase.
      b) Dosage: 50–100 mg po 2 times a day or tid.
      c) Side effects: hyperkalemia.
D. **Hair Removal**
   1. PhotoEpilation (laser) is more effective in women with dark hair and light skin.
   2. Topical treatment with eflornithine cream (Vaniqa) reduces hair growth.

Amenorrhea

I. Clinical Evaluation
A. History and physical exam
B. Laboratory Studies: Follicle stimulating hormone, TSH, prolactin, karyotyping. Measure serum testosterone and 17-OHP, if virilization is present.
C. Imaging: Pelvic ultrasound. MRI for CNS lesions.

II. Primary Amenorrhea
A. Primary amenorrhea is defined as lack of a menstrual period by age 14–15 in the absence of secondary sexual characteristics, or no menstrual period by age 16–17 years.
B. Causes of primary amenorrhea include gonadal failure (43%) due to 45 X. Congenital absence of uterus and vagina (15%) and constitutional delay (14%).
C. Clinical evaluation begins with genital examination and assessment of breast development.

III. Differential Diagnosis for Primary Amenorrhea
A. **Breast Present/Uterus Present**
   1. Secondary amenorrhea
   2. Imperforate hymen
   3. Transverse vaginal septum
   4. Vaginal agenesis
B. **Breast Present/Uterus Absent**
   1. Mullerian agenesis
   2. Androgen insensitivity

C. **Breast Absent/Uterus Present**
1. Constitutional delay
2. 45 X (Turner syndrome)
3. CNS tumor, trauma or infection
4. Congenital adrenal hyperplasia
5. Anorexia
6. Stress
7. Kallmann syndrome
8. Pure gonadal dysgenesis

D. **Breast absent/Uterus Absent**
1. 46 XY gonadal dysgenesis
2. 5 alpha-reductase, 17–20 desmolase, or 17 alpha-hydroxylase deficiency with XY karyotype

E. **Congenital Uterine and Vaginal Malformations**

F. **Imperforate Hymen**
1. Imperforate hymen is visible as a dark-blue bulging membrane. An abdominal mass may be palpable.
2. Treatment: A cruciate incision should be made from 2 to 8 o'clock and 10 to 4 o'clock.

G. **Transverse Vaginal Septum**: Ultrasound, MRI, and karyotyping are diagnostic. Treatment is resection. A vaginal dilator is used after surgery.

H. **Mullerian Agenesis**
1. 46 XX. Uterus, vagina, and fallopian tubes are absent or hypoplastic. Ovarian function and secondary sexual characteristics are normal
2. CT is used to exclude urinary tract and vertebral anomalies. Cardiac echo is used to exclude cardiac abnormalities and hearing tests if indicated
3. Oocyte retrieval and gestational surrogate may be used for fertility. Vaginal dilators are used to create a functional vagina.

IV. **Gonadal Dysgenesis**
A. **Turner Syndrome**
1. 45 X. Gonadal dysgenesis results in bilateral streak gonads, short stature, webbed neck, shield chest, and hypergonadotropic, hypoestrogenic amenorrhea. Turner syndrome is associated with autoimmune disorders and cardiovascular and renal anomalies.
2. Treatment of Turner syndrome is growth hormone starting at age 2–8 years. Estrogen and progestin at age 12–13 years.

B. **46 XY or 46 XX Gonadal Dysgenesis**
1. 46 XX or 46 XY causes streak gonads. Patients will reach normal height female with no sexual development. Normal female testosterone. Swyer syndrome is gonadal dysgenesis in 46 XY individuals.
2. Treatment is removal of gonads to prevent malignancy. Estrogen replacement should be provided.

V. **Androgen Insensitivity**
A. Androgen insensitivity is an X-linked recessive disorder. Patients have a 46 XY genotype, but female phenotype with normal female breasts and absent sexual hair. Patients have a short or absent vagina. Testosterone level is in the normal male range. Androgen insensitivity is caused by absence of the testosterone receptor
B. Intra-abdominal or inguinal testes should be removed after puberty.

VI. **Kallmann Syndrome** is a congenital GnRH deficiency, which causes hypogonadotropic hypogonadism, anosmia or hyposmia, and delayed growth and sexual development

VII. **Secondary Amenorrhea**
A. Secondary amenorrhea is an absence of periods for 6 months or no periods for 3 cycles in women who have had menses. Common causes of

secondary amenorrhea include chronic anovulation, hypothyroidism, hyperprolactinemia, and weight loss.

B. **Hypothalamic Amenorrhea**
   1. Hypothalamic amenorrhea is caused by stress, weight loss, anorexia, bulimia, excessive exercise, and lesions of the CNS.
   2. The treatment of hypothalamic amenorrhea is estrogen replacement.

C. **Hyperprolactinemia**

D. **Etiology**
   1. Causes of excessive prolactin hormone levels include prolactinoma, hypothyroidism, renal or hepatic failure, nipple massage, and pregnancy. The prolactin level declines to normal 6 months postpartum in nursing mothers.
   2. Medications associated with hyperprolactinemia include antipsychotics (risperidone), metoclopramide, antidepressants, antihypertensives, opiates, or H2 blockers.

E. **Pituitary Prolactinoma**
   1. Pituitary prolactinomas are microadenomas if less than 10 mm. Macroadenomas are larger than 10 mm.
   2. Prolactinomas cause oligomenorrhea, galactorrhea and infertility. Headache and visual changes result from mass compression

F. *Clinical Evaluation*
   1. If prolactin is elevated, assess pregnancy test, TSH, free T4, and metabolic panel.
   2. If amenorrheic, assess follicle stimulating hormone level to exclude ovarian failure.
   3. MRI is indicated in all patients with prolactinemia.

G. *Treatment*
   1. Asymptomatic microadenoma do not require treatment. Assess prolactin level and monitor response to dopamine agonist therapy.
   2. Dopamine agonists are the initial treatment of microadenoma or macroadenoma to restore euprolactinemia.
      a) Bromocriptine (Parlodel) 1.25–2.5 mg qhs. Increase by 1.25–2.5 mg weekly. Max 10 mg/day.
      b) Cabergoline (Dostinex) 0.25–0.5 mg po weekly. Increase by 0.25–0.5 mg weekly. Max 3 mg/week.
      c) Side effects include dizziness, nausea and vomiting, nasal congestion, and orthostatic hypotension. Cabergoline has fewer side effects.
      d) Transsphenoidal surgery or radiation is only indicated for a few patients who do not respond to medical therapy.

H. **Asherman Syndrome**
   1. Asherman syndrome is amenorrhea because of intrauterine scaring caused by uterine curettage or infection
   2. Diagnosis of Asherman syndrome is by hysteroscopy followed by an intrauterine pediatric Foley for 7 days. High dose estrogen is prescribed to stimulate endometrial growth.

I. **Spontaneous Premature Ovarian Failure**
   1. Premature ovarian failure is defined as spontaneous development of amenorrhea, elevated follicle stimulating hormone, and low estrogen before 40 years of age.
   2. Premature ovarian occurs in 1% of women.

J. **Clinical Evaluation**
   1. Ovarian failure is diagnosed by a follicle stimulating hormone of more than 30 mIU/mL. E2 is <50 pg/mL
   2. Adrenal, pancreas, thyroid, and parathyroid function should also be assessed.

3. Karyotyping is indicated if the patient is ≤30 years of age. Exclude fragile X permutation, which causes mental retardation, autism, and CGG gene repeats.
K. **Treatment** of premature ovarian failure is hormone replacement therapy and prevention of osteoporosis. Fertility is accomplished by in vitro fertilization.

Pediatric Gynecology

I. **Pediatric Pelvic Examination**
   A. The knee-chest position is the optimal position for pelvic examination of children.
   B. The vaginal mucus membrane of children is redder and thinner than the mucus membrane of an adolescent after puberty. The vaginal pH is normally neutral.
II. **Common Gynecologic Conditions**
   A. **Vulvovaginitis**
      1. Vulvovaginitis is the most common gynecologic disease. Only 25% of vaginal cultures grow an organism.
      2. A foreign body may cause bloody or foul-smelling discharge. Sexual abuse is suggested by trichomonas, gonorrhea, or Chlamydia. Some children may be colonized with Chlamydia at birth. HPV infection in children usually results from indirect, nonsexual transmission.
      3. Allergies, pinworms, and dermatitis can cause vulvovaginitis.
   B. **Treatment:**
      1. Infections should be treated. Sitz baths and reduce exposure to bubble bath and harsh soaps should be recommended.
      2. Topical estrogen cream with oral antibiotics may be prescribed for a maximum of 4 weeks.
   C. **Vaginal Bleeding** is rare before adolescence. Bleeding etiologies may include foreign bodies, neoplasia, precocious puberty, trauma, sexual assault, vulvovaginitis, urethral prolapse, bleeding disorders, lichen sclerosis, and Shigella.
   D. **Adhesive Vulvitis**
      1. Adhesive vulvitis causes the labia to appear fused into a thin vertical line.
      2. Treatment of adhesive vulvitis is topical estrogen cream 2 times a day, which usually causes the vulva to separate in 2 weeks.
   E. **Genital Trauma**
      1. Genital trauma often results from a straddle injury. Sexual abuse is also possible.
      2. Lacerations should be repaired and evaluate for injury to other pelvic organs. Exam under anesthesia is usually necessary.
   F. **Adnexal Mass**
      1. Adrenal masses usually present with lower abdominal pain or a palpable mass. The mass may torse, bleed, and rupture.
      2. Adnexal tumors in children are usually benign (75%). Benign teratoma is the most frequent tumor, and germ cell tumor is the most frequent malignancy. Germ cell tumor is assessed with inhibin, β-hCG, AFP, and LDH.
   G. **Puberty** consists of the physical and physiologic maturations that facilitate reproduction.
   H. **Tanner Staging**
      1. **Stage 1**
         a) Breasts are prepubertal. Only the papilla are elevated
         b) Pubic hair: None

2. **Stage 2**
   a) Breast budding occurs at 9.8 years
   b) Pubic hair is sparse. The long hair along the labia majora appears at 10.5 years
3. **Stage 3**
   a) Breasts have enlargement of glandular tissue, smooth contours at 11.2 years
   b) Pubic hair is coarse with curled hair on the mons at 11.4 years
4. **Stage 4**
   a) Breasts have a secondary mound of areola at 12.1 years
   b) Pubic hair is adult-type hair but hair is limited to mons at 12.0 years
5. **Stage 5**
   a) Breasts have a mature, smooth contour at 14.6 years
   b) Pubic hair is adult-type at 13.7 years

I. **Order of Changes:**
1. Breast development (thelarche)
2. Pubic hair and axillary hair growth (pubarche and adrenarche)
3. Bone growth spurt (peak height velocity)
4. Menstrual bleeding (menarche): average age 12.9 years
5. **Precocious Puberty** is the development of secondary sexual characteristics before 7 years of age in Caucasians or 6 years of age in African Americans, or menarche before age 8 years

J. **Classification of Precocious Puberty**
1. **GnRH-dependent precocious puberty** includes idiopathic precocity (74%) and CNS diseases (tumor, infection, trauma, and congenital anomalies).
2. **GnRH-Independent Precocious Puberty** includes ovarian cysts or tumors, McCune-Albright syndrome (polyostotic fibrous dysplasia, café au-lait spots, and endocrinopathies), congenital adrenal hyperplasia or adrenal tumors, and ectopic GnRH production.

K. **Clinical Evaluation**: Follicle stimulating hormone, luteinizing hormone, TSH, T4, testosterone, DHEAS, 17-alpha-hydroxyprogesterone, estradiol, brain MRI, and bone age survey.

L. **Treatment of Precocious Puberty**
1. Isolated premature thelarche or adrenarche usually regresses spontaneously.
2. GnRH analogues are indicated to treat true precocity to prevent short stature.

III. Delayed Puberty and Etiology
A. Hypogonadotropic hypogonadism due to constitutional delay is the cause of most cases at delayed puberty. Other etiologies include chronic diseases, malnutrition, pituitary tumor, craniopharyngioma, hyperprolactinemia, and Kallmann syndrome.
B. Hypergonadotropic hypogonadism results from gonadal dysgenesis and ovarian failure.

Benign Vulvar Diseases

I. Vulvovaginal Pruritus
A. Etiologies of vulvovaginal pruritus include infectious vaginitis, atrophic vaginitis, dermatitis, psoriasis, lichen sclerosus, lichen planus, lichen simplex chronicus, cancer, Paget disease, hidradenitis suppurativa, scabies, pediculosis pubis, and vulvodynia

II. Vulvar Dermatitis
A. Vulvar dermatitis is the most common skin condition.

B. Vulvar dermatitiscauses chronic lichenification of the vulva.

III. Treatment
  A. Mild cases are treated with 2.5% hydrocortisone or 0.5% triamcinolone daily for 2 weeks.
  B. Lichenification is treated with clobetasol, fluocinonide, or halobetasol 0.05% ointment daily for 4 weeks, then every other day for 2–4 weeks.
  C. Hydroxyzine 50–100 mg qhs is used to reduce pruritis.

IV. Lichen Sclerosus
  A. Atrophic disease occurs in all age groups and is most frequent in elderly patients.
  B. Vulva lichen sclerosus is associated with vulvar squamous cell cancer.
  C. Vulva or epithelium appears thin, atrophic, and white.
  D. Biopsy is needed to confirm the diagnosis.
  E. **Treatment of Lichen Sclerosus**: Clobetasol or halobetasol 0.05% ointment qhs 6–12 weeks, then 1–3 times a week.

V. Vulvodynia
  A. Vulvodynia is vulvar pain, including burning, stinging, or dyspareunia. The vulva has a normal appearance.
  B. Treatment of vulvodynia consists of antidepressants, topical estrogen, gabapentin or carbamazepine, topic lidocaine or EMLA, and precoital lubricant before intercourse.
  C. Surgery is reserved for localized vulvodynia.

VI. Bartholin Gland Abscess
  A. Bartholin glands are located at 4 and 8 o'clock position on the vaginal orifice. Duct obstruction leads to cyst or abscess formation.
  B. Large cysts may cause pain or dyspareunia.
  C. Treatment
    1. Bartholin gland abscesses are treated with incision and drainage and insert ion of Word catheter. The catheter should remain in place for 2–4 weeks. Antibiotics are indicated if cellulitis has developed.
    2. Marsupialization or excision is done for recurrent cysts or abscesses.

Menopause

Menopause is defined as 12 months of amenorrhea. The menopausal transition begins in the mid-to-late 40s with duration of 4 years and is characterized by menstrual irregularity. The median age of menopause is 50–52 years.

I. Menstrual Cycles During the Menopausal Transition
  A. The early menopausal transition is characterized by shortening of menstrual cycle. The follicle stimulating hormone is more than 10 mIU/ml
  B. Late menopausal transition is characterized by a cycle length of more than 42 days. Follicle stimulating hormone is greater than 30–40 mIU/ml

II. Hormone Replacement Therapy
  A. **Risks and Benefits of Hormone replacement therapy**
    1. Long-term hormone replacement therapy with combined estrogen and progestin is associated with a small increased risk of coronary heart disease, ischemic stroke, pulmonary embolism, breast cancer, and neurodegenerative disorder. Hormone replacement therapy decreases the risk of colon cancer and hip fracture.
  B. **Recommendations**
    1. Hormone replacement therapy should be avoided if the patient has a history of PE, deep vein thrombosis, or thrombophilia. Discontinue hormone replacement therapy if the patient has surgery, trauma, or prolonged immobilization.

2. Avoid hormone replacement therapy if the patient has a history of breast or endometrial cancer.
3. Hormone replacement therapy is effective in preventing and treating osteoporosis.
4. Women with premature menopause or surgical menopause should use hormone replacement therapy until 52 years of age.

III. Treatment of Menopausal Symptoms

A. Vasomotor symptoms include hot flashes. Dyspareunia results from vaginal atrophy.

B. **Vasomotor Symptoms**
1. Hot flashes are caused by an absence of estrogen.
2. Hormone replacement therapy is used to treat menopause-related symptoms at the time of menopause. The benefits of HRT declines in older women.

C. **Systemic Estrogen**
1. Systemic estrogen is prescribed if the patient has moderate to severe menopausal symptoms
2. Estrogen and progestin are prescribed if uterus is present.
3. Estrogen alone is prescribed after a hysterectomy.
4. Conjugated estrogen 0.45 or 0.3 mg/day, transdermal estradiol 0.025 or 0.014 mg/day, or oral estradiol 0.5 mg/day is prescribed.
5. Discontinuation should be considered after 12 month to 5 years of therapy.

D. **Selective serotonin-reuptake inhibitors and serotonin-norepinephrine reuptake inhibitors**
1. Venlafaxine (Effexor XR) 75 mg to 150 mg po qd
2. Paroxetine (Paxil CR) 25 mg po qd
3. Escitalopram (Lexapro) 10 or 20 mg po qd.

E. **Vaginal Atrophy**
1. Vaginal estrogen is more effective than systemic estrogen for vaginal dryness and dyspareunia. Progesterone is not needed when low-dose vaginal estrogen is used for genital atrophy.
2. Avoid vaginal estrogen if the patient has a history of breast cancer.
3. Common vaginal estrogen regimens:
   a) Conjugated estrogen cream 0.5 gram 1 to 3 times a week
   b) Vaginal tablet 10 µg twice a week.
   c) Vaginal ring 7.5 µg/day

F. **Commonly Used Agents for Hormone Replacement Therapy**
G. **Estrogen-Progestin**
1. **PremPro:** Conjugated estrogen and medroxyprogesterone acetate; 0.3mg/1.5mg, 0.45mg/1.5mg, 0.625mg/2.5mg, 0.625mg/5mg. 28-day EZ-Dial dispensers
2. **PremPhase**: Conjugated estrogen 0.625 mg in the initial 14 pills followed by conjugated estrogen 0.625mg/medroxyprogesterone acetate 5mg from day 15–28; 28-day EZ-Dial dispensers
3. **FemHRT**: Ethinyl estradiol /norethindrone acetate; 2.5 mcg/0.5 mg and 5 mcg/1 mg; 28-day blister pack
4. **Prefest**: Ethinyl estradiol 1 mg for 15 tabs and ethinyl estradiol/norgestimate 1 mg/0.09 mg for 15 tabs; 30-day blister pack
5. **Activella:** Ethinyl estradiol/norethindrone acetate; 1 mg/0.5mg and 0.5 mg/0.1 mg
6. **Angeliq:** Ethinyl estradiol/drospirenone 1 mg/0.5 mg

H. **Estrogen only**
1. **Premarin:** Conjugated estrogen 0.3, 0.45, 0.625, 0.9, and 1.25 mg
2. **Congest**: Conjugated estrogen 0.3, 0.45, 0.625, 0.9, and 1.25 mg
3. **Cenestin**: Synthetic conjugated estrogens; 0.3, 0.45, 0.625, 0.9, and 1.25 mg

4. **Enjuvia**: Synthetic Conjugated estrogens; 0.3, 0.45, 0.625, 0.9, and 1.25 mg
5. **Estrace**: Estradiol 0.5 mg, 1 mg, 2 mg
6. **Gynodiol**: Estradiol 0.5 mg, 1 mg, 1.5 mg, 2 mg
7. **Femtrace**: Estradiol 0.45 mg, 0.9 mg, 1.8 mg
8. **Ogen**: Estropipate 0.75, 1.5, 3, and 6 mg
9. **Ortho-Est**: Estropipate 0.75, 1.5, 3, and 6 mg
10. **Menest**: Esterified estrogens 0.3, 0.625, 1.25, and 2.5 mg

I. **Progestins**
1. **Aygestin**: Norethindrone acetate; 5 mg
2. **Prometrium**: Micronized progesterone 100 mg and 200 mg
3. **Provera**: Medroxyprogesterone acetate 2.5 mg, 5 mg, and 10 mg
4. **Amen**: Medroxyprogesterone acetate 2.5 mg, 5 mg, and 10 mg

J. **Estrogen-Testosterone**
1. **Covaryx HS**: Esterified estrogens 0.625 mg and methyltestosterone 1.25
2. **Covaryx**: Esterified estrogens 1.25 mg and methyltestosterone 2.5 mg
3. **EEMT HS**: Esterified estrogens 0.625 mg and methyltestosterone 1.25 mg
4. **EEMT**: Esterified estrogen 1.25 mg and methyltestosterone 2.5 mg
5. **Syntest DS**: Esterified-estrogens 1.25 mg/methyltestosterone 2.5 mg
6. **Syntest HS**: Esterified-estrogens 0.625 mg/methyltestosterone 1.25 mg

K. **Estrogen-Progesterone Patch**
1. **Combi-Patch:** Estradiol/norethindrone. 0.05 /0.14 mg/day and 0.05/0.25 mg/day. Apply twice a week.
2. **Climara Pro**: Ethinyl estradiol/levonorgestrel, 0.045/0.015 mg/day. One patch per week

L. **Estrogen-Only Patch**
1. **Alora**: Estradiol patch, 0.025 mg, 0.05 mg, 0.075 mg, 0.1 mg /24h. Twice a week
2. **Climara:** Estradiol patch, 0.025 mg, 0.0375 mg, 0.05 mg, 0.06 mg, 0.075 mg, or 0.1 mg/24h. Once a week
3. **Esclim**: Estradiol patch, 0.025 mg, 0.0375 mg, 0.05 mg, 0.075 mg, 0.1 mg/24h, twice a week
4. **Estraderm**: Estradiol patch, 0.05 mg, 0.1 mg/24h, twice a week
5. **FemPatch**: Estradiol patch, 0.025 mg, once a week
6. **Menostar**: Estradiol patch, 0.014 mg/24h, once a week
7. **Vivelle and Vivelle-Dot**: Estradiol patch, 0.05 mg, 0.0375 mg, 0.05 mg, 0.075 mg, 0.1 mg/24h, twice a week
8. **Estrogen Gel**: Apply to arm, shoulder, thigh, or abdomen once a day at the same time each day. Avoid breasts
9. **Divigel 0.1%**: Estradiol gel, 0.25, 0.5, and 1 g/day
10. **Elestrin 0.06%**: Estradiol gel, 1.7 and 0.87 g/day
11. **EstroGel 0.06%**: Estradiol gel, 1.25 g/day
12. **Estrogen Emulsion**: Apply to both thighs and calves every morning. Avoid breasts
13. **Estrasorb**: Estradiol daily dose: two 1.74 g pouches per day

M. **Estrogen Spray**
1. **Eva Mist**: Estradiol 1.53 mg /spray, 1–3 sprays to inner forearm daily

N. **Estrogen Injection**
1. **Delestrogen**: Estradiol valerate 10 mg/ml, 20 ml/ml, 40 mg/ml. 10–20 mg IM every 4 weeks for vasomotor symptoms

2. **Depo-Estradiol**: Estradiol cypionate 5 mg/ml; 1–5 mg IM every 4 weeks

O. **Vaginal Estrogen for Vaginal Atrophy**

1. **Premarin**: Conjugated estrogen 0.625 mg/gram. One tube contains 42.5 g cream; 0.5, 1, 1.5, or 2 g vaginally a day
2. **Estrace**: Ethinyl estradiol cream, 0.1 mg ethinyl estradiol/1 g cream in 42.5 g tube, 2–4 g/day for 1–2 weeks, then 1–2 g/d for 1–2 weeks. Maintenance: 1 g 1–3 times/week
3. **Estring**: Ethinyl estradiol vaginal ring, 7.5 mcg/24h. Replace every 90 days.
4. **Femring**: Ethinyl estradiol vaginal ring, 0.05 mg/day and 0.1 mg/day. Replace q 3 months.
5. **Vagifem**: Ethinyl estradiol 10 mcg tablet, 1 tab qd for 2 weeks, then 1 tab twice weekly.

Osteoporosis

I. **Definition**
   A. Normal bone mineral density is a T score of ≥ –1
   B. Osteopenia (low bone mass) is a T score between –1 and –2.5
   C. Osteoporosis is a T score ≤ –2.5
   D. **T-score** is the number of standard deviations from the mean of the peak normal bone mineral density.
   E. **Z-score** is the number of standard deviations from the mean bone mineral density. Used in younger women. Diagnostic evaluation for etiologies other than postmenopausal bone loss is recommended if the Z-score is ≤ –2.0 SD.

II. **ACOG Indications for Bone Mineral Density Testing**
   A. All women ≥65 years
   B. Postmenopausal women less than 65 years with any risk factor:
      1. Medical history of a fragility fracture
      2. Body weight less than 127 lb
      3. Medical causes of bone loss (medications or diseases)
      4. Parental history of hip fracture
      5. Current smoker
      6. Alcoholism
      7. Rheumatoid arthritis

III. **Dual-energy X-ray Absorbtiometry (DEXA)**
   A. DEXA of hip and spine is the standard test for osteoporosis. Screening should be every 2 years in the absence of new risk factor.

IV. **Treatment**
   A. **Preventive Measures**: Balanced diet, adequate calcium and vitamin D, regular weight-bearing exercise, smoking cessation, moderation of alcohol, and fall prevention
   B. **Institute of Medicine Recommendations**
      1. Calcium: 1,300 mg for adolescents (age 9 to 18 years); 1,000 mg for women aged 19 to 50 years; 1,200 mg for women aged >51 ears
      2. Vitamin D: 600 IU/day for women aged ≤70 and 800 IU/day for women aged ≥71 year for bone health.
   C. **Indications for Pharmacologic Treatment in Postmenopausal Women**
      1. Prior osteoporotic vertebral of hip fracture.
      2. T score ≤ –2.5 SD at the femoral neck, total hip, or spine
      3. T score –1 to –2.5 SD at the femoral neck, total hip, or spine and a 10-year probability of a hip fracture ≥3%, or a 10-year probability of a major osteoporosis-related fracture ≥20%.

D. **Pharmacologic Agents for the Treatment of Osteoporosis**
  1. **Bisphosphonates**
     a) Bisphosphonates reduce bone resorption and are the first line therapy for postmenopausal osteoporosis. Bisphosphonates reduce vertebral fracture by 70% and reduce the nonvertebral fracture rate by 35%.
     b) Bisphosphonates are usually discontinued after 5 to 10 years.
     c) Esophageal and gastric irritation is common. Bisphosphonates should be taken on an empty stomach and remain upright for at least 30 min to prevent esophagea irritation.
     d) The serum calcium should be monitored, and renal function should be assessed before initiating bisphosphonates.
       (1) Alendronate (Fosamax) 5 mg po qd or 35 mg weekly for prevention of vertebral fractures; 10 mg qd or 70 mg weekly for treatment of osteoporosis
       (2) Risedronate (Actonel): 5 mg po qd or 35 mg weekly for prevention and treatment; 150 mg once a month for fracture prevention. Risedronate delayed release (Atelvia) 35 mg weekly.
       (3) Ibandronate (Boniva) 2.5 mg po qd, 150 mg once a month, or 3 mg IV every 3 months for treatment of osteoporosis. Oral doses are used for prevention of vertebral fractures.
       (4) Zoledronic acid (Reclast): 5 mg IV annually.
  2. **Selective Estrogen Receptor Modulators**
     a) Raloxifene (Evista) : 60 mg po qd for prevention of and treatment of vertebral fracture.
     b) SERMs are used for breast cancer prevention in postmenopausal women.
     c) SERMs are associated with an increased risk of venous thromboembolism, stroke, and vasomotor symptoms.
  3. **Estrogen**: Estrogen is an option for osteoporosis treatment and fracture prevention for 5 years or less if early menopause when other treatments for osteoporosis are not appropriate.
  4. **Parathyroid hormone (Recombinant Human PTH 1-34)**
     a) PTH is an anabolic agent, which enhances bone density.
     b) Teriparatide (Forteo) is approved for the treatment of osteoporosis in postmenopausal women at high-risk of fracture for no longer than 24 months. PTH is used for severe osteoporosis or after failure of bisphosphonates.
  5. **Denosumab (Prolia)**
     a) Denosumab inhibits osteoclast by binding to the RANK ligand. Denosumab is indicated for the treatment of postmenopausal women with osteoporosis at high risk for fracture, or after failure of other osteoporosis therapies.
     b) 60 mg every 6 months as a subcutaneous injection.
E. **Follow-up** DEXA is usually done after 1 to 2 years of treatment. If bone mineral density is improved or stable, repeat DEXA is not needed.

Female Sexual Dysfunction

I. **Sexual Desire Disorders**
   A. Hypoactive sexual desire disorder (HSDD) is a persistent or recurrent deficiency, or absence of sexual thoughts, fantasies, and/or desire for or receptivity to, sexual activity, which causes significant distress.
   B. Sexual aversion disorder is a persistent or recurrent aversion to genital contact with a partner that results in distress or interpersonal difficulty.

    C. **Sexual Arousal Disorder** is the inability to complete sexual activity with adequate lubrication, resulting in significant distress or interpersonal difficulty. SAD is often caused by medical conditions and selective serotonin-reuptake inhibitors.

    D. **Orgasmic Disorder** is a persistent or recurrent delay in or absence of orgasm after a normal excitement phase.

II. Sexual Pain Disorders
    A. Dyspareunia is recurrent or persistent genital pain with intercourse that is not due to absence of lubrication or vaginismus.

    B. Vaginismus is involuntary spasm of the outer third of vagina, which interferes with intercourse.

III. Evaluation of Female Sexual Dysfunctions
    A. Emotional factors and personal relationship

    B. Depression, anxiety, diabetes, and hypothyroidism
       1. Antihypertensive: thiazide diuretics, ACE inhibitors, and calcium channel blockers
       2. Tricyclic antidepressants and selective serotonin-reuptake inhibitors

    C. Assess for history of sexual abuse, drug use, and alcoholism.

IV. Treatment of Female Sexual Dysfunctions
    A. **Sex Therapy**
       1. Sex devices: clitoral vibrators are available. The EROS clitoral vacuum device is approved for female sexual dysfunctions.

    B. **Hormonal Therapy**
       1. Estrogen is indicated for women with genital atrophy to improve vaginal blood flow and lubrication.
       2. Transdermal testosterone may be effective for short-term (6-month) treatment of hypoactive sexual desire disorder. Androgen therapy may cause hirsutism, acne, virilization, and cardiovascular disease.
       3. Bupropion (Wellbutrin 300 mg SR) is effective in premenopausal women with hypoactive sexual desire disorder.

Hysterectomy

The most common indications for hysterectomy are uterine leiomyoma, endometriosis, and uterine prolapse.

I. ACOG Guidelines on Prophylactic Bilateral Salpingo-oophorectomy
    A. *Factors Favoring Oophorectomy*
       1. Increased risks for ovarian cancer because of a family history or genetic testing, such as BRCA1 and BRCA2 mutation or HNPCC. Risk-reducing bilateral salpingo-oophorectomies are usually done at age 35–40 after childbearing.
       2. Adjuvant therapy for breast cancer in premenopausal women with hormone-sensitive cancer
       3. Bilateral ovarian neoplasms
       4. Severe endometriosis
       5. Ovarian cancer prevention in postmenopausal women
       6. Pelvic inflammatory disease or bilateral tuboovarian abscess

    B. *Factors Favoring Ovarian Preservation*
       1. Premenopausal status
       2. Concerning impact on sexual function, libido, and quality of life in young women
       3. Premenopausal women with osteopenia, osteoporosis or risk factors for osteoporosis

II. Type of Hysterectomy
A. **Total Abdominal Hysterectomy**
1. Most common method of hysterectomy. Easy to perform. Higher morbidity than other types of hysterectomy.
2. Reserved for the patients who are not candidates for transvaginal hysterectomy.
B. **Transvaginal Hysterectomy**
1. Preferred method of hysterectomy
2. Low complications, quick recovery, short hospital stay, and invisible incision
3. Limiting factors include undescended and immobile uterus and narrow vagina
C. **Laparoscopic-Assisted Vaginal Hysterectomy** has a more rapid recovery, less pain, and better cosmetic result than total abdominal hysterectomy.
D. **Total Laparoscopic Hysterectomy** requires greater laparoscopic experience. More complications.
E. **Total Robotic Hysterectomy** is often used for hysterectomy, myomectomy, sacrocolpopexy, and tubal reanastomosis. Robotic hysterectomy improves 3-D vision and instrument dexterity.

Perioperative Care

I. Preoperative Care
A. **Preoperative Laboratory Tests**
B. **Pregnancy test**
C. **Urinalysis**
D. **Hemoglobin/hematocrit**
E. **Type and screen**
F. **Coagulation tests (INR/aPTT)**
G. **Creatinine**
H. **Electrolytes**
I. **Chest X-ray**
J. **Electrocardiogram**

II. Medications
A. Medications are usually taken with 30 ml of water on the morning of surgery.
B. If patient is on NPO after surgery, use intravenous, transdermal or transmucosal medication.
C. *Medications with thrombogenic potentials (oral contraceptives, hormone replacement therapy, and SERMs)*
1. For minor procedures, continue these medications perioperatively.
2. For high-risk surgery, thrombogenic medications should be stopped 4–6 weeks prior to surgery. Consider heparin for venous thromboembolism prophylaxis if patient is on oral contraceptive or hormone replacement therapy at the time of surgery.
D. *Nonsteroidal anti-inflammatory drugs* should be stopped at least 3 days prior to surgery.
E. *Antiplatelet agents*
1. Aspirin: stop aspirin 7–10 days prior to surgery if the patient takes aspirin for chronic pain. Continue aspirin if the aspirin is being taken for inhibition of platelet aggregation after a coronary stent, CBAG or peripheral arterial surgery.
2. Other antiplatelet agents should continue.

F. **Corticosteroids**
1. Patients taking prednisone in a dose of 5 mg or less or any dose for less than 3 weeks, should take the same doses perioperatively.
2. If high-dose prednisone has been used for more than 3 weeks, supplemental corticosteroids should be given to prevent adrenal crisis:
   a) For minor procedures, give 25 mg of hydrocortisone IV on the day of surgery.
   b) For hysterectomy and higher stress gynecological procedures, give 50 mg of hydrocortisone IV on the day of surgery and taper to usual dose.

G. **Warfarin**
1. For major surgery, the INR should be less than 1.5. Stop warfarin 5 days before surgery. For minor surgery, the INR should be 1.5 to 2.0 and stop warfarin 3 days before surgery.
2. For urgent surgery, give vitamin K 1–5 mg IV or fresh frozen plasma or prothrombin complex concentrate before to surgery.
3. Warfarin should be restarted 12–24h after surgery.

H. **Heparin and low molecular weight heparins**
1. Stop heparin 4–6 hours prior to surgery and stop low molecular weight heparin 24 hours before surgery.
2. Restart heparin or low molecular weight heparin 24 hours after surgery.

III. **Gynecological Procedures and Antibiotic Prophylaxis Regimens**
A. **Hysterectomy and urogynecologic procedures**
1. Cefazolin (Ancef) 1g IV f before anesthesia induction. Give 2 g if weight >100 kg or 220 lb. A second dose of cefazolin may be given if surgery is more than 3 hours or if EBL is ≥1,500 ml

B. **Immediate Hypersensitivity to Penicillin:**
1. Clindamycin 600 mg IV plus gentamicin 1.5 mg/kg IV or
2. Metronidazole (Flagyl) 500 mg IV plus gentamicin 1.5 mg/kg IV or
3. Ciprofloxacin, levofloxacin or moxifloxacin 400 mg IV or
4. Aztreonam 1 g IV

C. **Elective surgical abortion or D&E**
1. Doxycycline 100 mg 1 hr before the procedure and 200 mg PO after procedure or
2. Metronidazole (Flagyl) 500 mg po 2 times a day for 5d

IV. **Thromboembolism Prophylaxis**
A. **Risk Factors**
1. Surgery, trauma, immobility, malignancy, previous venous thromboembolism, older age, pregnancy and the postpartum period, estrogen oral contraception or hormone replacement, SERMs, myeloproliferative disorders, and thrombophilias.

B. **Method of Venous Thromboembolism Prophylaxis**
1. Graduated compression stocking and intermittent pneumatic compression should be place before surgery and continued until hospital discharge.
2. Low-dose unfractionated heparin: 5,000 units SC, q8–12h starting 1–2h before surgery and continue until discharge.
3. Low molecular weight heparins:
   a) Dalteparin 5,000 units, or enoxaparin (Lovenox) 40 mg SC, starting 12 hours before surgery and daily until discharge.
   b) Fondaparinux (Arixtra) , 2.5 mg SC once a day, can be given 6–8h after surgery.
   c) If unable to give low molecular weight heparin 12h before surgery, give first dose low molecular weight heparin 6–12h postoperatively.

C. **Low-Risk Surgeries** of less than 30 min, age less than 40 year, and no risk factors do not require prophylaxis
D. **Moderate-Risk Surgeries and Prophylactic Options**
    1. Surgeries less than 30 min with additional risk factors. Surgery less than 30 min aged 40–60 years. Major surgery less than 40 years
    2. Prophylaxis: low-dose unfractionated heparin q12h, low molecular weight heparin (dalteparin 2,500 u or enoxaparin 40 mg), graduated compression stockings, or intermittent pneumatic compression
E. **High-Risk Surgeries and Prophylactic Options**
    1. Surgery <30 min in patients more than 60 years or age 40–60 years with additional risk factors. Major surgery in patients more than 40 years or with additional risk factors.
    2. Prophylaxis: low-dose unfractionated heparin q8h, low molecular weight heparin, or intermittent pneumatic compression
F. **Prophylactic Options for Highest-Risk Surgeries**
    1. Prophylaxis: low-dose unfractionated heparin q8h, low molecular weight heparins, or intermittent pneumatic compression or graduated compression stockings plus low-dose unfractionated heparin or low molecular weight heparins.
    2. Continue prophylaxis for 2–4 weeks after surgery.

V. Postoperative Care
A. Pain Management
    1. **Intravenous Opioids and NSAIDs**
        a) Morphine 1–5 mg every 2–3 hours prn. Hydromorphone (Dilaudid) 0.2–1 mg q2–3h prn. Fentanyl 10–100 mg q2–3h prn.
        b) Ketorolac (Toradol): Given 15–30 mg q4–6h, limit use to less than 4 days.
    2. **Patient Controlled Analgesia**
        a) Morphine
           (1) Bolus: 1–10 mg
           (2) Maintenance: 1–3 mg, 6–10 min lockout
           (3) Hourly max: 15 mg
        b) Hydromorphone (Dilaudid)
           (1) Bolus: 0.2–2 mg
           (2) Maintenance: 0.2–0.6 mg, 6–10 min lockout
           (3) Hourly max: 3 mg
        c) Fentanyl
           (1) Bolus: 10–100 mcg
           (2) Maintenance: 10–30 mcg, 6–10 min lockout
           (3) Hourly max: 200 mcg
    3. **Common Oral Analgesics**
        a) Percocet-5 (acetaminophen 325 mg and oxycodone 5 mg), 1–2 tabs every 3–6 hours as needed
        b) Vicodin (acetaminophen 500 mg and hydrocodone 5 mg), 1–2 tabs every 3–6 hours
        c) Oxycodone 5, 15, or 30 mg po every 4–6 hours
        d) Oxycodone sustained release (OxyContin) 10, 20, 40, or 80 mg every 12 hours as needed
        e) Morphine controlled release (MS Contin) 30, 60, 100, or 200 mg every 8–12 hours
        f) Ibuprofen 200, 400, 600, or 800 mg every 4–6 hours
B. Pelvic Cellulitis and Abscess
    1. Pelvic cellulitis and abscess will cause a fever on post-op day 3–5 with pain in lower abdomen, which is tender to palpation.
    2. **Treatment of Pelvic Cellulitis and Abscess**
        a) CT with contrast will demonstrate a fluid collection and pelvic in-flammation.

      b) Small abscesses respond to IV Metronidazole (Flagyl) 1 gm IV q12h and Piperacillin-tazobactam (Zosyn) 3.375 gm IV q4-6h.

      c) Large abscesses may need drainage. Abscess can be drained vaginally or percutaneously.

C. **Postoperative Ileus**
   1. The colon will regain function after 2-3 days. Flatus signals recovery of normal bowel function.
   2. The patient may have gas pain, abdominal distension, nausea, and vomiting.

D. **Clinical Features of Postoperative Ileus**
   1. Postoperative ileus causes postop, diffuse discomfort or pain resulting from abdominal distension. Bowel sounds are absent
   2. X-ray pattern: Bowel is diffusely distended. Gas is visible throughout GI tract

E. **Clinical Features of Bowel Obstruction**
   1. Bowel obstruction results from adhesions and usually occurs 5 days after surgery with intermittent abdominal cramping. High-pitched bowel sounds are audible
   2. X-ray patterns: Proximally dilated loops of bowel with air-fluid levels. Distal bowel does not have gas.

F. **Treatment of Postoperative Ileus**: Supportive care: NPO, IV hydration, correction of electrolyte deficits, ambulation, minimize narcotic use, and laxative suppository or enema.

VI. Wound Complications

A. **Wound infections** usually occur between day 5 to day 10 with pain, fever, and tachycardia. Incisions are erythematous, tender, fluctuant, and indurated.

B. *Treatment of Wound Infections*
   1. Open the wound, drain the exudate, debride the edge, and irrigate the wound with normal saline.
   2. Use wet-to-dry gauze dressing to pack the wound. Change the dressing 2–3 times a day.
   3. Give antibiotics if the wound is erythematous and warm.

C. **Hematoma or Seroma**
   1. Hematoma or seroma occur more frequently with transverse incisions resulting in pain and drainage of bloody fluid from the wound
   2. Small seromas are managed expectantly. Large hematomas should be opened, drained, and packed.

VII. Post-Op Instructions

A. For minor procedures, such as dilation and curettage and laparoscopy, a follow-up visit should be scheduled in 2 weeks.

B. For hysterectomy or other major surgeries, follow-up should be scheduled at 2 and 6 weeks. Perform a complete pelvic exam at 6 weeks. Staples should be removed on post-op 5–7 days for vertical incision.

C. Avoid lifting heavy objects more than 15 lb

D. No intercourse until for 6-weeks.

VIII. Post-operative Orders

    Admit to:

    Diagnosis:

    Condition: stable, guarded.

    Vitals: q8h

    Allergies: NKA

    Activity: up to chair, ambulate QID.

    Nursing: intermittent pneumatic compressions, incentive spirometry 10/hr while awake, Foley to gravity, I/Os, daily weight, or O_2 by NC to maintain saturations >95%

    Diet: NPO, regular, or as tolerated

IV Fluid: DSNS and rate
Medications: pain medications, antiemetics, antibiotics, deep vein
thrombosis prophylaxis
Laboratory Studies: CBC, metabolic panel
Special studies: X-ray, CT
Call resident for:

IX. Brief Operative Note

Pre-op diagnosis:
Post-op diagnosis:
Procedure:
Surgeon and Attending:
Assistant:
Anesthesia:
Fluids: Crystalloid and blood products
Estimated blood loss:
Drains:
Specimen:
Operative findings:
Complications:
Disposition:

Infertility

Reproductive Physiology

I. **Age and Fertility**
   A. Germ cells decrease in number after 16–20 weeks gestational age: 6 million germ cells are present at 16–20 weeks of gestational age, 2 million at birth, 500,000 at onset of puberty, and 25,000 at age 37–38.
   B. The fertility of a woman peaks between 20–24 years of age, then declines slowly after 30 years, more rapidly after 35 years, and declines very rapidly after 37 years. By 40 years, fertility is severely reduced.

II. **Menstrual Cycles**
   A. Regular cycles are a sign of ovulatory cycles. Amenorrhea or oligomenorrhea is a sign of anovulation.
   B. Irregular cycles are common in the first 2 years after menarche and 3 years before menopause.

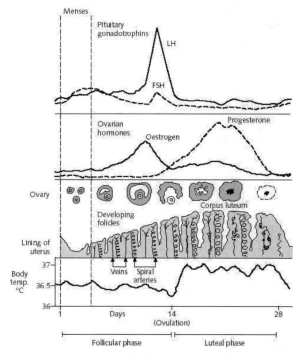

Figure: The menstrual cycle

III. **Fertility Window**
   A. Cycle fecundability is the probability that a single cycle will result in pregnancy. The fecundability is 20% for a young, fertile couple.
   B. The cumulative pregnancy rates in a normal couple is 57% at 3 months, 72% at 6 months, 85% at 1 year, and 93% at 2 years.
   C. Normal sperm survive 3–5 days. Oocytes survive only 12–24 hours after ovulation. The fertility window is 6 days (5 days prior to ovulation and the day after ovulation).
   D. The highest probability of conception occurs if intercourse takes place 1–2 days before ovulation.

IV. **Timed Intercourse for Infertility Couples**
   A. Observing the change in vaginal discharge is a simple method for timing intercourse. Ovulation causes cervical glands secrete copious mucus, which is clear, stretchy, and slippery (Spinnbarkeit mucus).

Infertility Evaluation

I. **Definition and Etiologies**
   A. Infertility is defined as failure to conceive after 1 year of unprotected intercourse. 7% of women are infertile. Women over the age of 35 years should be evaluated after 6 months of failure to conceive with unprotected intercourse.
   B. Causes of infertility include ovulatory dysfunction (17.6%), tubal disease (23%), endometriosis (7%), male factor (24%), unexplained (25%), and luteal phase defect, cervical factor, and uterine defect (3%).

II. **Clinical Evaluation**
   A. **HPI:** Assess the patient's and partner's reproductive history, length of infertility, coitus frequency, and lubrication use.
   B. **Past GYN:** menarche, menstrual cycle regularity, flow, dysmenorrhea, and molimina, history of sexually transmitted diseases, past contraception, and last menstrual period
   C. **PMH:** thyroid problems, weight gain or loss, galactorrhea, and history of chemotherapy or radiation
   D. **Past Surgical History:** Pelvic or abdominal surgery, e.g., cervical, ovarian or uterine surgery, appendectomy, or endometriosis ablation
   E. **Social History:** tobacco, alcohol or drug use, diet and exercise, and stress
   F. Medications

III. **Physical Examination**
   A. Weight
   B. Signs of anorexia: thinning or drying of the hair, lanugo, dry skin, yellow palms, swollen salivary glands, and dental erosions.
   C. Signs of androgen excess: excessive hair on face, chest and abdomen; acne and temporal balding
   D. Thyroid and breast: assess for enlarged thyroid glands or nodules and galactorrhea
   E. Abdomen and pelvis: assess for pelvic inflammatory disease, leiomyoma, and endometriosis

IV. **General Screening Laboratory Studies**
   A. TSH, prolactin, Pap, blood type, Rh factor, antibody screening, rubella, RPR, chlamydia, gonorrhea, hepatitis B and C, and HIV

V. **Semen Analysis**
   A. Normal semen analysis excludes out male factor infertility. The semen analysis should be repeated if the initial test was abnormal; 1 to 3 days

of abstinence is adequate. Prolonged abstinence more than 10 days decreases sperm motility and fertility.

B. Low sperm count should be evaluated with a measurement of testosterone level.

C. **Normal Semen Parameters**
   1. Semen volume: 1.5 million/mL (1.4–1.7)
   2. Sperm concentration: 15 million/mL (12–16)
   3. Total Number: 39 million/mL (33–46)
   4. Total progressive and nonprogressive motility: 40% (38–42)
   5. Progressive motility: 32% (31–34)
   6. Normal forms: 4% (3.0–4.0)
   7. Vitality: 58% (55–63)

VI. Ovulation Tests

A. **OTC Ovulation Prediction Kits (LH Kits)**
   1. LH kits monitor midcycle luteinizing hormone release with urine dipsticks. The luteinizing hormone surge normally lasts 48–50 hours. Begin testing 1 to 2 days before the expected surge.
   2. For women with regular 28-day cycle, start testing on day 10.
   3. LH becomes positive 24–38 hours before ovulation. The couple should have intercourse on the day of and day after a positive LH test.

B. **Basal Body Temperature:** Measure and chart temperature each morning before arising. Ovulation has a biphasic pattern with a nadir on the day of ovulation and an increase after ovulation.

C. **Midluteal Serum Progesterone**
   1. Assess progesterone one week prior to expected menses or 7–8 days after the luteinizing hormone surge.
   2. A serum progesterone level >3 ng/ml indicates ovulation has occurred.

VII. Pelvic Ultrasound

A. Ultrasound detects fibroids, uterine septum, and ovarian cysts.

B. Ultrasound can measure the antral follicle count and ovarian volume can be used to predict ovarian reserve.

VIII. Hysterosalpingogram

A. HSG delineates the anatomy of the uterus and tubes, and HSG detects tubal occlusion

B. HSG should be scheduled on cycle day 5–11, between day 2 to 5 after the end of menses.

IX. Ovarian Reserve Tests

A. **Serum Markers**
   1. Follicle stimulating hormone, estradiol (E2), and inhibin are measured on cycle day 2 to 4. FSH is abnormal if >12 IU/L.
   2. Anti-Müllerian hormone evaluates ovarian reserve and can be drawn at any point in the menstrual cycle. An AMH of less than 0.6 indicates severe ovarian impairment.

B. **Hysteroscopy is used to** diagnose and treat intrauterine pathology.

C. **Combined Laparoscopy and Hysteroscopy**
   1. Laparoscopy and hysteroscopy are definitive tests for tubal factors, which are seen on HSG.
   2. Chromotubation is injection of a dilute indigo carmine dye through a cannula attached to the cervix. Chromotubation evaluates tubal patency.

Treatment of Female Infertility

I. **Recommendations for Infertility Couples**
   A. Stop smoking and discontinue drug use.
   B. Maintain body mass index between 20 and 25.
   C. Limit alcohol to less than 5 drinks/week and limit caffeine to less than 250 mg/day.
   D. Decease heavy aerobic exercise

II. **WHO Classification of Ovulatory Dysfunction**
   A. Group I–Hypogonadotropic hypogonadism: decreased GnRH, low or normal follicle stimulating hormone and luteinizing hormone, and low estrogen. Etiologies include weight loss, excessive exercise, anorexia, Kallmann syndrome, and CNS lesions. Accounts for 10% of cases.
   B. Group II–Eugonadotropic anovulation: normal follicle stimulating hormone, estrogen, and prolactin. Frequently seen in polycystic ovarian syndrome. Characterized by amenorrhea or oligomenorrhea with elevated androgen. Accounts for 70% of cases.
   C. Group III–Hypergonadotropic-hypogonadism (ovarian failure): amenorrhea with elevated follicle stimulating hormone. Occurs in Turner syndrome and premature ovarian insufficiency. 10% of cases.
   D. Hyperprolactinemia: 10% of cases.

III. **ESHRE/ARSM Consensus on Infertility Caused by Polycystic Ovarian Syndrome**
   A. 5% of weight loss prior to intervention is advised if overweight.
   B. First-line therapy: clomiphene citrate
   C. Second-line therapy: exogenous gonadotropins.
   D. Third-line therapy: in vitro fertilization

IV. **Clomiphene Citrate (Clomid, Serophene)**
   A. Clomiphene is a selective estrogen receptor modulator, which triggers GnRH and follicle stimulating hormone secretion by depleting estrogen receptors in the pituitary and hypothalamus.
   B. Induces ovulation in 60% of patients. Cycle fecundity is 15% if ovulation occurs. Cumulative pregnancy rate is 30% and multiple pregnancy rate 5%.
   C. Young and amenorrheic women have high success rate. Response is lower with increased age, BMI, and hyperandrogenemia.
   D. Side effects: hot flushes, bloating and pelvic discomfort, and vomiting, headache, and visual complaints.

V. **Clomiphene Protocol**
   A. Start clomiphene at any time if the patient has had no recent uterine bleeding and a documented negative pregnancy test. Or start clomiphene 50 mg on cycle day 2, 3, 4, or 5 for 5 days.
   B. Ovulation usually occurs 5 to 10 days after the last dose of clomiphene. Test for ovulation with luteinizing hormone kit starts 3 days after the last clomiphene. Use vaginal ultrasound to evaluate ovarian follicles.
   C. Begin daily or every-other-day intercourse 3 days after last clomiphene until 1–2 days after ovulation.
   D. Document ovulation with basal body temperature or a progesterone level 1 week after positive luteinizing hormone testing. If progesterone is less than 10, increase clomiphene by 50 mg/day for next cycle.
   E. Check urine pregnancy test before starting the next cycle.
   F. Increase clomiphene to 100 mg in next cycle if ovulation failed. Clomiphene maximum dose is 250 mg/day.

VI. Additional Measures

    A. Intrauterine insemination on the day or day after luteinizing hormone surge

    B. Monitor follicle growth with serial ultrasound starting day 10–12. Give hCG 50–10,000 IU IM when the follicle is 18–25 mm. Perform intrauterine insemination 36 hours after hCG injection.

VII. Exogenous Gonadotropins

    A. Need intensive monitoring with serial serum estradiol levels and vaginal ultrasound.

    B. Risk of multiple pregnancy and ovarian hyperstimulation syndrome. Withholding hCG trigger if more than 4 follicles >14 mm.

VIII. Ovarian HyperstimulationSyndrome

    A. OHS is a complication of ovulation induction with exogenous gonadotropins. Increased capillary permeability results in a fluid shift from the intravascular to the extravascular spaces.

    B. Severe ovarian hyperstimulation syndrome can cause ascites, pleural effusion, electrolytes disturbances, hemoconcentration, oliguria, and thromboembolism.

IX. Treatment of Non-Ovulatory Etiologies of Infertility

    A. **Endometriosis.** Severe endometriosis may cause infertility.

        1. Medical therapy for endometriosis reduces pain but does not improve the fertility rate.

        2. Endometriosis has a good in vitro fertilization success rate. Endometriosis is associated with a low oocyte fertilization rate.

        3. Laparoscopic surgery with excision or ablation does not improve fertility in mild endometriosis. Endometrioma ≥4 cm are removed; however, removal of endometriomas can reduce ovarian reserve.

Assisted Reproductive Technologies

Assisted reproductive technologies are associated with a twin gestation rate of 29% and a high-order gestation rate of 2%.

I. Terminology

    A. Assisted reproductive technologies includes in vitro fertilization, intracytoplasmic sperm injection, assisted hatching, and donor eggs.

    B. In vitro fertilization combines an egg and sperm. IVF is the most frequent assisted reproductive technology.

    C. Intracytoplasmic sperm injection is injection of a single sperm into a mature oocyte.

II. In Vitro Fertilization Steps

    A. **Ovarian Stimulation**

        1. Therapy with 150 IU FSH/day is started shortly after spontaneous or progesterone-induced bleeding and continued until a dominant follicle (>10 mm) is seen on transvaginal ultrasonography. The dose is then decreased to 112.5 IU/day followed by a further decrease to 75 IU/day 3 days later, which is continued until hCG 250 mcg is administered to induce ovulation.

        2. Serial estradiol and pelvic ultrasound are performed after the start of the stimulation.

    B. **Oocyte Retrieval**: Ultrasound guided follicular aspiration is performed 34–36 hours after the hCG injection.

    C. **In Vitro Fertilization, Embryo Culture and Transfer**

        1. Oocytes are inseminated 4 hours after retrieval and zygotes are cultured for 3 days.

2. Preimplantation genetic diagnosis may be used to identify and exclude a genetic disease.

III. Luteal Phase Support with Progesterone

A. Daily progesterone lateral phase support should start on the day of or the day after oocyte retrieval.

B. Vaginal progesterone: 8% progesterone gel (Crinone) 90 mg qd or micronized progesterone (Prometrium) 200 to 600 mg/day or vaginal insert (Endometrin) 100 mg 2 times a day or 3 times a day.

C. Progesterone IM: 50 mg/day

D. Perform serum β-hCG 9–12 days after the embryo transfer.

Pelvic Floor Disorders

Urinary Incontinence

Urinary incontinence occurs in 25% of reproductive-age women, 40% of postmenopausal women, and 50% of women in nursing homes.

I. **Definition**
   A. Stress incontinence causes involuntary loss of urine on exertion, coughing, or sneezing.
   B. Urge incontinence causes involuntary loss of urine with urgency.
   C. Mixed urinary incontinence is characterized by stress and urge incontinence.

II. **Clinical Evaluation**
   A. Determine the number of times patient voids during the day and during the night. Evaluate the severity of leakage.
   B. During the last 3 months, have you leaked urine?
   C. Did you leak urine when you cough, sneeze, lift, or exercise? Did you leak urine when you have the urge to empty your bladder, but you cannot get to the toilet fast enough?
   D. Which one occurs most often, leaking with stress or leaking with urge?

III. **Pelvic Examination**
   A. External genitalia: Assess for vulvar, vaginal, and urethral atrophy and irritation.
   B. Neurological exam: Assess bulbocavernosus reflex.
   C. Speculum and bimanual exam: evaluate vagina while straining. Assess urethral hypermobility and pelvic prolapse.
   D. Evaluate levator strength by having the patient perform a Kegel's contraction.

IV. **Office Testing**
   A. Urinalysis and urine culture to rule out urinary tract infection.
   B. Q-tip test demonstrates urethral mobility.
   C. Postvoid residual with urine catheter or bladder ultrasound excludes urinary retention.
   D. Cough stress test will demonstrate stress incontinence when the patient coughs with a full bladder.
   E. Cystometrogram uses a straight catheter, bulb syringe, and normal saline to assess bladder volume and detrusor instability.

V. **Indications for Urodynamic Tests**
   A. Uncertain diagnosis
   B. Plan surgical intervention
   C. Possible neurologic disease
   D. Overflow incontinence

VI. **Behavioral Therapy**
   A. Avoid bladder irritants, such as caffeine, tea, and alcohol.
   B. Timed voiding and smoking cessation
   C. Decrease fluid intake after 7 pm.
   D. Bladder retraining at increasing intervals to improve bladder volume and decrease bladder spasm.

VII. **Pelvic Floor Muscle Exercises:** Kegel exercises, vaginal cone, vaginal pessary, electrical simulation, and biofeedback.

VIII. Medications for Urge and Mixed Incontinence

    A. Anticholinergics cause dry mouth, constipation, and blurred vision. Anticholinergics are contraindicated in narrow-angle glaucoma.

    B. **Antimuscarinic Medications for Urinary Incontinence**

        1. Oxybutynin (Ditropan): initial dose 2.5 mg po 2 times a day–tid. Maximum 10 mg 2 times a day or tid

        2. Oxybutynin extended-release (Ditropan XL): start 5 mg po qd. Increase by 5 mg every week. Max 30 mg per day

        3. Oxybutynin patch (Oxytrol): 1 patch (5 mg) twice weekly

        4. Oxybutynin gel 10% (Gelnique): Apply once daily to the skin.

        5. Tolterodine (Detrol): 2 mg po 2 times a day.

        6. Tolterodine extended-release (Detrol LA): 4 mg po qd

        7. Trospium (Sanctura): 20 mg po 2 times a day

        8. Trospium (Sanctura XR): 60 mg po qd

        9. Solifenacin (Vesicare): 5 or 10 mg po qd.

        10. Darifenacin (Enablex): 7.5 or 15 mg po qd

        11. Fesoterodine (Toviaz): 4–8 mg po qd

        12. Imipramine (Tofranil): 25–75 mg po qhs

IX. Surgical Treatment of Stress Incontinence

    A. **Midurethral Sling is the** gold standard for stress urinary incontinence

    B. *Retropubic Sling— Transvaginal Tape (TVT)*

        1. Transvaginal tape has a success rate of 81% vs. 80% with Burch procedure.

        2. Blind passage of the trocar through retropubic space may cause injuries to bladder, major blood vessels, bowel, ureter, or urethra.

        3. Intra-operative cystoscopy is performed.

    C. *Trans-Obturator Tape*

        1. Placed trans-obturator tape inside the vagina, coming out through the obturator foramen or starting from the groin area, passing through obturator foramen, then coming out in the vagina.

        2. Transobturator tape prevents major vascular, ureteral, and bowel injury and reduces the risk of bladder injuries.

    D. *Comparison Between transvaginal tape and Transobturator tape*

        1. Objective success rate: 80% in transvaginal tape group and 77% in transobturator tape group

        2. Voiding dysfunction requiring surgery: 2.7% in transvaginal tape group vs. 0% in transobturator tape

        3. Neurologic symptoms: 4.0% in transvaginal tape group vs. 9.4% in transobturator tape group

X. Surgical Treatment of Urge Incontinence

    A. **Botulinum Toxin Type A (Botox) Injection**

        1. Inject Botox (100 to 200 units) into the posterior bladder wall by cystoscopy.

        2. Improvement occurs in 60% and effective for 1 year.

        3. Major complication is increased postvoid residual, and self-catheterization may be needed.

    B. **Bulking Agents for Intrinsic Sphincter Deficiency (ISD)**

        1. ISD is a severe form of stress incontinence. Treatment of ISD includes transvaginal tape and transobturator tape procedures.

        2. Periurethral injection of bovine collagen, carbon beads and calcium hydroxylapatite may be indicated in women with excessive surgical risks.

Pelvic Prolapse

Pelvic prolapse develops in 25% of women due to vaginal delivery, aging, and elevated intraabdominal pressure.

I. Terminology for Pelvic Prolapse
   A. Uterine prolapse is prolapse of the uterus and cervix into the vagina
   B. Cystocele is prolapse of bladder into the vagina
   C. Rectocele is prolapse of rectum into the vagina
   D. Enterocele is herniation of bowel into the vagina
   E. Vaginal vault prolapse is prolapse after hysterectomy.

II. Staging of Pelvic Organ Prolapse
   A. **Stage 0:** No prolapse is demonstrated.
   B. **Stage 1:** The most distal portion of the prolapse is more than 1 cm above the hymen.
   C. **Stage 2:** The most distal portion of the prolapse is ≤1 cm proximal to or distal to the hymen.
   D. **Stage 3:** The most distal portion of the prolapse is more than 1 cm below the hymen but protrudes no further than 2 cm less than the total vaginal length.
   E. **Stage 4:** Complete eversion of the total length of the lower genital tract.

III. Clinical Evaluation
   A. Assessment includes severity of prolapse, leaking of urine with stress or urgency, difficulty with urination or recurrent urinary tract infections, anal incontinence, and dyspareunia.
   B. **Pelvic Exam**
      1. Inspect vaginal wall with single speculum blade.
      2. Examine the patient in lithotomy and standing positions, and induce prolapse with Valsalva.
      3. Perform rectovaginal exam to evaluate enterocele, posterior wall defect, pelvic muscle, and strength of anal sphincter.

IV. Nonsurgical Treatment
   A. Kegel exercises.
   B. **Pessaries** are effective, economical, and noninvasive. A Pessary should be offered as the first line therapy.
   C. Start with size 4 ring-type pessary. One end of the pessary is placed in the posterior fornix and the other end is placed behind the symphysis.

V. Surgery
   A. **Preoperative Counseling**
      1. Bowel and sexual function may not improve after surgery. Surgery may cause dyspareunia.
      2. Surgical repair is done after childbearing.
   B. **Cystocele or Cystourethrocele**
      1. **Paravaginal Repair or Site-Specific Repair**
         a) The vagina is attached to the arcus tendineus. Repair can be accomplished abdominally, laparoscopically, or vaginally.
      2. **Apical Defect and Vaginal Vault Prolapse**: Perform hysterectomy if uterus is present.
         a) **Sacrocolpopexy**
            (1) Suspend the vagina or uterus to the anterior longitudinal ligament of the sacrum with graft material.
            (2) Advantages: restores vagina to normal anatomic position, preserve vaginal length, and has a low recurrence.
         b) **Uterosacral Ligament Suspension**
            (1) Suspend the vaginal cuff to the bilateral uterosacral ligaments.

        (2) Intra-operative cystoscopy is performed to identify ureteral obstruction.

    c) **Sacrospinous Ligament Fixation**: Suspends the vaginal apex to the sacrospinous ligaments.

    d) **Iliococcygeal Suspension**: Suspend the vaginal apex to the iliococcygeus muscle and fascia. Easy to perform.

C. **Posterior Compartment Defect (Rectocele)**

  1. **Posterior Colporrhaphy or Colpoperineorrhaphy:** Plicate the levator ani in the midline. Excessive trimming of the vaginal mucosa and perineal skin can cause vaginal narrowing.

  2. **Site-Specific Repair**: The fascial defects can be identified by placing a finger in the rectum. Repair fascial defects.

Gynecologic Oncology

Gestational Trophoblastic Diseases

Gestational trophoblastic diseases include hydatidiform mole, invasive mole, choriocarcinoma, and placental site trophoblastic tumor.

I. Hydatidiform Mole
   A. 90% of complete moles are caused by duplication of a haploid sperm (absent maternal chromosomes); 10% are because of fertilization of an empty ovum by 2 sperm.
   B. Hydatiform moles will cause abnormal vaginal bleeding and high b-hCG. Ultrasound confirms the diagnosis by absence of fetus and edematous villi in complete moles.
   C. Partial moles present as a missed or incomplete abortion. Ultrasound shows abnormal sac or malformed fetus with a hydropic placenta. Diagnosis is made after curettage.
   D. **Pretreatment Evaluation**
      1. CBC, type and screen (RhoGAM is given if Rh negative), chest X-ray, metabolic panel, and hCG
      2. TSH and free T4 if indicated
   E. **Treatment**
      1. Suction D&E is the preferred method of evacuation under ultrasound guidance with IV oxytocin.
      2. Hysterectomy is performed for women who do not desire future fertility.
      3. Twin gestations complicated by GTD are treated with suction curettage if termination is desired. No intervention if continue the pregnancy is desired. Vaginal bleeding, preeclampsia, preterm labor or fetal demise may occur.
   F. **Post-Treatment Follow-up**
      1. **Contraception and hCG Monitoring**
         a) Birth control is administered for 1 year.
         b) Assess hCG weekly until normal for 3 consecutive weeks, then monthly for 6 months, then yearly for 1–3 years
         c) False-positive hCG may result from nonspecific protein interference and heterophile antibodies. Urine hCG will be negative.

II. Gestational Trophoblastic Neoplasia
   A. **Risk Factors for Postmolar Gestational Trophoblastic Neoplasia**
      1. Pre-evacuation hCG >100,000
      2. Uterine size greater than gestation dates
      3. Theca lutein cysts >6 cm
   B. **FIGO Diagnostic Criteria for Postmolar GTN**
      1. Plateau of hCG lasts for four measurements over a period of 3 weeks or longer
      2. hCG level rise of >10% above baseline for three values over 2 weeks
      3. hCG level remains elevated for 6 months or more
      4. Pathological diagnosis of choriocarcinoma
      5. Presence of metastatic disease
   C. Diagnosis of Metastases
      1. Chest X-ray diagnoses lung metastases.
      2. Liver metastases may be diagnosed by CT scan.

3. Brain metastases may be diagnosed by CT scanning.
    D. **FIGO Staging Criteria for Gestational Trophoblastic Neoplasia**
       1. Stage I: Disease confined to uterus
       2. Stage II: Extends outside uterus but limited to genital structure
       3. Stage III: Metastases to lung
       4. Stage IV: Involves other metastatic sites
    E. **Gestational Trophoblastic Neoplasia Types**
    F. **Invasive Mole**
       1. Trophoblastic tissue penetrates into the myometrium.
       2. Invasive moles occur in 10–17% of hydatidiform moles, resulting in vaginal bleeding after molar pregnancy. Diagnosed by persistent elevation of hCG.
       3. Invasive moles regress spontaneously.

III. **Choriocarcinoma**
    A. Choriocarcinoma usually presents with late postpartum bleeding.
    B. Choriocarcinoma develops from trophoblastic tissue.
    C. Metastases to lung, liver, brain, pelvis, vagina, spleen, intestine, and kidney.

IV. **Placental Site Trophoblastic Tumor**
    A. Placental site trophoblastic tumor is a rare disease, which causes vaginal bleeding and uterine enlargement. PSTT causes low levels of hCG and HPL. Metastases occur late.
    B. PSTT is treated with hysterectomy and is resistant to chemotherapy.
    C. **Chemotherapy**
       1. **Low-Risk** *Gestational Trophoblastic Neoplasia*
          a) Gestational trophoblastic neoplasia has a 90% remission rate with methotrexate or actinomycin D.
          b) Monitor serum hCG weekly, and administer chemotherapy until the hCG normalizes, and then give at least 1 course after hCG normalization.
          c) Hysterectomy is used to shorten the treatment course if the patient does not desire fertility.
       2. *Regimens for Low-Risk Gestational Trophoblastic Neoplasia*: 5-Day Regimen: methotrexate 0.4 mg/kg IV or IM qd for 5 days every 2 weeks. Or actinomycin D 10–13 ug/kg IV for 5 days every 2 weeks
       3. **EMA/CO Regimen for High-Risk Metastatic** *Gestational Trophoblastic Neoplasia*
          a) **Day 1:** Etoposide 100 mg/m2, Methotrexate 100 mg/m2 followed by 200 mg/m2 IV infusion over 12 hours, and Actinomycin D 0.5 mg IV
          b) **Day 2:** Etoposide 100 mg/m2 IV infusion, actinomycin D 0.5 mg IV, and folinic acid 15 mg IV/IM/PO every 6 hours for 4 doses.
          c) **Day 8:** Cyclophosphamide 600 mg/m2 IV and vincristine (Oncovin) 1 mg/m2 IV
          d) Start next cycle on day 15, and repeat 2–3 cycles after hCG normalizes.

Cervical Cancer

Cervical cancer has a median age of diagnosis of 48 years and median age at death is 57 years. The 5-year survival rate for stage IA1 cervical cancer is 97%, IA2 95%.

I. **Risk Factors**
    A. HPV infection is the primary risk factor for cervical cancer. HPV 16 accounts for 50% of all cervical cancers and HPV 18 causes 30% of can-

cers. Other high-risk HPV types are HPV 31, 33, 35, 39, 45, 51, 52, and 58.

II. Diagnosis of Cervical Cancer
   A. Cervical cancer is asymptomatic at early stage. Abnormal vaginal bleeding and excessive vaginal discharge are common.
   B. Exophytic lesions are the most frequent type.

III. Cervical Biopsy
   A. Diagnosis is by cervical biopsy, endocervical curettage, and conization.
   B. Visible lesions should be biopsied. Pap smear can be negative in 50% of cases.

IV. Histology of Cervical Cancer
   A. Adenocarcinoma 25%
   B. Adenosquamous carcinoma 3–5%.

V. Staging
   A. Cervical cancer staging is with physical exam, colposcopy, hysteroscopy, cystoscopy, proctoscopy, X-ray of lung and skeleton, IVP, and cone biopsy.
   B. CT, MRI, and PET are widely used for planning treatment.
   C. FIGO Staging of Cervical Cancer
   1. **Stage 0:** Carcinoma in situ or CIN 3
   2. **Stage I**: Cancer is confined to the uterus.
      a) *Stage IA*
         (1) Invasive carcinoma that can be diagnosed only by microscopy.
         (2) Maximal depth of stromal invasion is less than 5 mm and width is less than 7 mm.
         (3) Vascular space, venous, or lymphatic involvement should not change the staging.
         (4) IA1: Stromal invasion less than 3 mm and extension less than 7 mm
         (5) IA2: Stromal invasion >3 mm but less than 5 mm. Extension less than 7 mm
      b) *Stage IB*
         (1) All gross lesions are designated stage 1B. Clinically visible lesions limited to the cervix or preclinical cancers greater than stage IA.
         (2) IB1: Visible lesions <4 cm
         (3) IB2: Visible lesions >4 cm
   3. **Stage II**: Cervical carcinoma invades beyond the uterus, but not to the pelvic wall or to the lower third of the vagina.
      a) *Stage IIA*
         (1) No obvious parametrial involvement
         (2) IIA1: Visible lesions <4 cm
         (3) IIA2: Visible lesions >4 cm
      b) *Stage IIB*: Obvious parametrial involvement.
   4. **Stage III**: Carcinoma extends to pelvic wall and/or involves the lower third of vagina, and/or results in hydronephrosis or nonfunctioning kidney.
      a)*IIIA*: Tumor involves lower 1/3 of the vagina, with no extension to the pelvic wall.
      b)*IIIB:* Extension to pelvic wall. All cases with hydronephrosis or a nonfunctioning kidney are included.
   5. **Stage IV:** Cancer spread to adjacent or distant organs.
      a) *IVA*: Extends beyond the true pelvis or involves the mucosa of the bladder or rectum.
      b) *IVB*: Distant metastasis, including peritoneal spread or para-aortic lymph nodes.

VI. Treatment
A. Stage IA1
1. Diagnosed with cold knife cone or LEEP. Conization with clear surgical margins and a negative ECC is adequate treatment for young women who desire fertility.
2. Repeat cone should be performed if the margins or ECC indicate dysplasia or microinvasion before proceeding to simple hysterectomy.

B. Stage IA2
1. Type II/modified radical hysterectomy or radical trachelectomy and pelvic lymph node dissection
2. **Incidental Cervical Cancer on Simple Hysterectomy Specimen**
   a) Stage IA1 requires no further treatment. Stage IA2, requires re-operation to remove parametrium and upper third of vagina, and perform pelvic lymph node dissection.

C. Stage IB1 and Non-bulky IIA
1. Both RH with complete pelvic lymph node dissection and radiation therapy are equally effective.
2. Radiation therapy is indicated for all patients. Radiation may damage the bladder, small intestine, and rectosigmoid colon. Vaginal stenosis may be prevented with a vaginal dilator after radiation therapy.
3. RH eliminates primary disease, prevents chronic damage to the bladder, bowel, and vagina by the radiation.
4. High-risk factors for recurrence include positive lymph nodes, positive surgical margins, parametrial extension, large size of primary tumor, deep stromal invasion, lymph-vascular space invasion, and high-grade histology.
5. Postoperative radiation is indicated for high-risk factors.

D. Stage IB2 and Bulky IIA
Cisplatin-based chemoradiation is recommended.

E. Stage IIB to IVA
Cisplatin-based chemoradiation is recommended with external pelvic radiation then brachytherapy with concurrent weekly cisplatin 40 mg/m2 to a total dose of 200 mg/m2.

F. Stage IVB
Cisplatin and radiation are used for local control. Cisplatin and topotecan are used for systemic therapy.

G. Surveillance
Symptoms and signs of recurrence include abdominal and pelvic pain, leg pain or edema, vaginal bleeding or discharge, urinary symptoms, cough and weight loss

H. Cervical Cytology
1. Perform Pap smear once a year
2. Treatment: abnormal cytology occurs in one third of patients during follow-up. ASC-US or LSIL may be followed without colposcopy unless abnormalities persist. ASC-H and HSIL are evaluated with colposcopy.

Uterine Cancer

Endometrial cancer is the most frequent gynecologic cancer with a lifetime incidence of 2%. Median age at diagnosis is 63 years. Median age at death is 73 years.

I. Risk Factors for Uterine Cancer:
A. Exposure to unopposed estrogen, obesity, chronic anovulation, diabetes, hypertension, post-menopause, tamoxifen, obesity, diabetes, low parity, early menarche, and late menopause
1. Estrogen-related tumors are usually low-grade, superficially invasive endometrioid cancers. Estrogen-unrelated tumors are usually papil-

lary serous or clear cell tumor, deeply invasive and metastatic and occur in older women.
2. The risk of endometrial cancer is decreased by oral contraceptives and hormone replacement therapy with continuous estrogen-progestin.

B. 5-year survival rate: IA 91%, IB 91%, IC 85%, IIA 83%, IIB 74%.

II. Diagnostic Evaluation

A. Indications for Evaluation
1. Postmenopausal bleeding includes exogenous estrogen (30%), atrophic endometritis/vaginitis (30%), cancer (15%), endometrial or cervical polyps (10%), and endometrial hyperplasia (5%).
2. Postmenopausal pyometra or endometrial cells on a Pap
3. Perimenopausal menorrhagia or metrorrhagia
4. Premenopausal patients with abnormal uterine bleeding.

B. Office Endometrial Biopsy
1. Endometrial biopsy is the first step in evaluating abnormal uterine bleeding
2. The Pipelle device detects 95% of endometrial cancer in post-menopausal women and 90% in premenopausal women.

C. Transvaginal Ultrasound
1. Post-menopausal thickness of endometrial strip: atrophic 3.4 mm, hyperplasia 9.7 mm, and endometrial cancer 18 mm. Endometrial strip <4 mm is low risk, 4–7 mm equivocal, and >8 mm suspicious.
2. Endometrial biopsy is advised if the endometrial strip is >4 mm in postmenopausal women with bleeding.
3. Endometrial biopsy may not be required if the endometrial strip is less than 4 mm.

D. Dilation and Curettage is indicated if endometrial biopsy is negative but there is a high suspicion of malignancy with continued unexplained bleeding.

E. Endometrial Hyperplasia
1. Endometrial hyperplasia is excessive proliferation of endometrial glands. Nuclear atypia increases the risk of endometrial cancer.
2. Classifications of endometrial hyperplasia and risk of progressing to cancer: simple hyperplasia 1%, complex hyperplasia (adenomatous) 3%, atypical simple hyperplasia 8%, and atypical complex hyperplasia 29%.

III. Treatment of Hyperplasia with Atypia
A. Hysterectomy is curative
B. Fertility-sparing treatment of endometrial hyperplasia is megestrol (Megace) 40 mg 2 times a day to QID with an endometrial biopsy every 3 months.

IV. Treatment of Hyperplasia with No Atypia
A. Medroxyprogesterone (Provera) 20 mg/day for 10–14 days each month with endometrial biopsy in 3–6 months
1. If endometrial biopsy is normal or atrophic, continue Provera 10 mg/days for 10 days each month.
2. If hyperplasia is persistent, give high dose progestins then repeat endometrial biopsy.

V. Endometrial Cancer
A. Preoperative Evaluation
1. History and physical exam.
2. CBC, metabolic panel, urinalysis, and CA 125.
3. CT of pelvis and abdomen, cystoscopy, and sigmoidoscopy.

B. Surgical Staging includes hysterectomy, bilateral salpingo-oophorectomy, pelvic and paraaortic lymph node dissection, and resection of disease.

C. **FIGO and TNM Surgical Staging of Endometrial Carcinoma**
D. **Stage I:** Tumor confined to corpus uteri
   1. **Stage IA:** Tumor is limited to endometrium or invades less than 50% of myometrium
   2. **Stage IB:** Tumor invades more than 50% of myometrium
E. **Stage II:** Tumor invades stromal connective tissue of the cervix, but does not extend beyond uterus
F. **Stage III:** Local and/or regional spread
   1. IIIA: Tumor invades the serosa and/or adnexa
   2. IIIB: Tumor spreads to the vagina or adjacent to the uterus
   3. IIIC1: Metastases to pelvic lymph nodes
   4. IIIC2: Metastases to para-aortic lymph nodes
G. **Stage IVA:** Tumor invasion of bladder and/or bowel mucosa
H. **Stage IVB**
   1. Distant metastasis to inguinal lymph nodes, intraperitoneal disease, lung, liver or bone
   2. Grades: degrees of histopathologic differentiation
   3. G1: ≤5% of nonsquamous or non-morular solid tumor; G2: 6–50% of solid tumor; G3: >50% of solid tumor
I. **Postoperative Treatment and Adjuvant Therapy**
   1. Risk factors for recurrence and poor prognosis include advanced age (≥60), papillary serous and clear carcinoma, high tumor grade and myometrial penetration, vascular space invasion, positive peritoneal or cervical cytology, large tumor, high nuclear grade, and tumor aneuploidy
   2. Patients with stage IA and grade 1 or 2 disease do not need adjuvant therapy.
   3. Vaginal brachytherapy can be used to reduce local recurrence in early stage cancer.
   4. External pelvic radiation can be used for early stage, high risk endometrial cancer or extrauterine disease confined to the lymph nodes and adnexa.
   5. Patients with advanced stage cancers and recurrent cancers are treated with chemotherapy.

Ovarian Cancer

I. **Epithelial Ovarian Cancer**
   A. Epithelial ovarian cancer is the second most frequent gynecologic cancer, the most common cause of GYN cancer deaths, and the fifth-ranking cause of all cancer death. Lifetime risk is 1.3%. Median age at diagnosis is 63.
   B. 90% of ovarian malignancies are epithelial ovarian cancer.
   C. Risk factors for ovarian cancer include family history of ovarian cancer, BRCA 1 and BRCA 2 carriers, Lynch II syndrome, history of breast cancer, White race, low parity, infertility, early menarche, late menopause, and hormone replacement therapy with estrogen for >10 years
   D. Protective factors: oral contraceptives, breastfeeding, full term pregnancy, multiparity, tubal ligation, and hysterectomy with oophorectomy
   E. 5-year survival rate for ovarian cancer IA is 89.6%, IB 86%, IC 83%, IIA 70.7%, IIB 65.5%, IIC 71%, IIIA 46.7%, IIIB 41.5%, IIIC 32.5%, IV 19%
II. **Clinical Manifestations and Diagnosis**
   A. 75% ovarian cancer is diagnosed at stage III-IV. Ascites, pelvic mass, and GI metastasis occur in advanced ovarian cancer.
   B. **Early Symptoms**
      1. Bloating

2. Pelvic or abdominal pain
3. Difficulty eating or early satiety
4. Urgency or urinary frequency

C. **Tumor Markers**
1. CA 125 is a glycoprotein, which is elevated in >80% ovarian cancer. CA 125 is nonspecific for ovarian cancer. CA 125 is also elevated in breast, endometrial, lung and pancreatic cancer. CA 125 is increased in endometriosis, cirrhosis and pelvic inflammatory disease
2. CA 125 is useful follow-up marker for ovarian cancer
3. CEA and CA 19–9 are elevated in mucinous and endometrioid cancers
4. Human epididymis protein (HE4) is used for monitoring ovarian cancer progression and recurrence.

D. **Preoperative Workup**
1. Laboratory Evaluation: CBC, metabolic panel, and CA 125
2. CT of chest, abdomen and pelvis
3. If ovarian metastases are due to a Krukenberg tumor, perform colonoscopy, gastrointestinal endoscopy, and mammogram.

E. **FIGO Staging for Primary Carcinoma of the Ovary**
1. **Stage I:** Growth limited to the ovaries
   a) **IA:** Cancer limited to one ovary
   b) **IB:** Involve both ovaries
   c) **IC:** Tumor limited to one or both ovaries, but with one of the following:
      (1) Surface of one or both ovaries involved with tumor
      (2) Ruptured capsule
      (3) Ascites containing malignant cells
      (4) Washings of peritoneal cavity is positive for malignant cells
2. **Stage II:** Growth involving one or both ovaries with pelvic extension
   a) **IIA:** Extension and/or metastases to the uterus and/or tubes
   b) **IIB:** Extension to other pelvic tissues
   c) **IIC:** Tumor of either stage IIA or IIB, but with capsule ruptured, tumor on ovarian surface, malignant cells in ascites or peritoneal washings.
3. **Stage III**
   a) Tumor involving one or both ovaries with peritoneal implants outside the pelvis and/or positive retroperitoneal or inguinal nodes. Superficial liver metastasis is stage III. The tumor is limited to the true pelvis, but with malignant extension to small bowel or omentum.
      (1) **IIIA:** Tumor limited to the true pelvis with negative nodes but with microscopic seeding of abdominal peritoneal surfaces
      (2) **IIIB:** Tumor of one or both ovaries. Implants to abdominal peritoneal surfaces ≤2 cm in diameter. Nodes are negative.
      (3) **IIIC:** Abdominal implants are less than 2 cm in diameter and /or positive retroperitoneal or inguinal nodes
4. **Stage IV:** Distant metastasis. If pleural effusion with positive cytology is designated as stage IV. Liver metastasis is stage IV.

III. **Treatment**

A. **Treatment Based on Staging and Histology**
1. Histology types of epithelial ovarian cancer: papillary serous 75%, mucinous 10%, endometrioid 10%, clear cell, undifferentiated, and transitional cell 5%.
2. Stage IA or IB with grade 1 histology: surgical staging
3. Stage IA or IB with grade 2 or 3 and stage IC: staging and chemotherapy

      4. Stage II-IV: Total abdominal hysterectomy-bilateral salpingo-oophorectomy, debulking, and chemotherapy

B. **Surgery**

    1. Staging procedures for early stage cancer includes 1) cytologic evaluation of ascites or peritoneal washing; 2) examination and biopsy of the peritoneum of diaphragm, abdomen, and pelvis; 3) pelvic and para-aortic lymph node sampling; 4) Total abdominal hysterectomy-bilateral salpingo-oophorectomy and omentectomy; 5) appendectomy is performed for mucinous tumors.

    2. Debulking of advanced cancer increases survival.

C. **Standard Chemotherapy Regimen:** IV paclitaxel, followed by carboplatin every 21 days for 6 cycles

Operative Dictations

Cesarean Section

Name of Patient:
Patient Identification Number:
Date of Surgery:
Pre-op Diagnosis: (1) Term pregnancy at 39 weeks and 6 days; (2) Nonreassuring fetal heart rate tracing
Post-op Diagnosis: Same
Procedure: Primary low transverse cesarean section
Surgeon:
Assistant:
Attending:
Anesthesia: Epidural
EBL: 500 ml
Intravenous Fluid: 1000 ml
Urine Output: 300 ml
Specimen: Placenta sent to Pathology
Complication: None
Findings: Female infant in vertex position. Apgar 8/9. Weight 3,500 grams. Normal uterus, tubes, and ovaries
Indication and Consent

During labor the fetal heart rate pattern demonstrated late decelerations. Oxygen, left lateral position, and discontinuation of Pitocin did not improve the decelerations. Cesarean section was advised. The patient understood that the risks of cesarean section include visceral or vascular injury, infection, blood loss and need for transfusion, and reoperation. The patient stated an understanding and desired to proceed.

Procedure

The patient was taken to the operating room where epidural anesthesia was found to be adequate. Two grams of cefazolin (Ancef) were given. She was prepared and draped in the dorsal supine position with a leftward tilt. A Pfannenstiel skin incision was carried down to the fascia with a Bovie. The fascia was incised and extended laterally, and the inferior fascia was grasped with Kocher clamps. The rectus muscle and pyramidalis were dissected off sharply with Mayo scissors. The superior aspect of the fascia was elevated with a Kocher, and the rectus muscle was dissected off. Hemostasis was achieved with the Bovie. The rectus muscle was separated in the midline to the pubic symphysis. Pre-peritoneal fatty tissue was bluntly dissected to expose the peritoneum. The peritoneum was determined to be free of adherent bowel and entered with scissors. The peritoneal incision was extended superiorly and inferiorly to the bladder reflection with visualization of the bladder.

A bladder blade was inserted and vesicouterine peritoneum identified. Intraabdominal survey revealed scant, clear peritoneal fluid. The vesicouterine peritoneum was opened with scissors and the bladder flap was developed. The bladder blade was repositioned to retain the bladder out of the operative field. The lower uterine segment was incised with a scalpel. An Allis clamp was used to rupture the amniotic sac and clear fluid was observed. The uterine incision was extended bluntly.

The fetus presentation was cephalic. The fetal head was elevated out of pelvis. After the head was brought into the incision, gentle fundal pressure was applied. The infant was delivered and the mouth and nose were suctioned with a bulb. The cord was clamped and cut, and the infant was handed to the pediatrician. The placenta was delivered intact and IV oxytocin was initiated. The uterus was then exteriorized, and the uterine incision was closed with a running locking 2–0 Monocryl suture. The ovaries and tubes were normal. The uterus, tubes, and ovaries were then returned to the abdominal cavity. The uterine incision was reinspected and good hemostasis was observed.

The peritoneum was closed with running 4–0 Monocryl suture, and the fascial layer was closed with 2–0 PDS loop suture. The skin was closed with subcuticular 4–0 Monocryl suture. The patient tolerated the procedure well. All the counts were correct times two. The patient was taken to the recovery room in a stable condition.

Vacuum-assisted Vaginal Delivery

Date of Delivery:
Pre-op Diagnosis: (1) Term pregnancy; (2) Prolonged second stage labor
Post-op Diagnosis: Same
Procedure: Vacuum-assisted vaginal delivery
Surgeon:
Assistant:
Attending:
Anesthesia: Epidural
EBL: 300 ml
Complications: None
Findings: Female infant, weight 3,500 grams. Apgar 7 at 1 minute and 8 at 5 minutes. Second degree midline laceration
Indications and Consent
The 21-year-old G1P0 at 40 weeks pushed for more than 3 hours after complete cervical dilation. The perineum appeared edematous. The fetal head was in direct occiput anterior position at 2+ station. Pelvis was felt to be adequate for vaginal delivery and the fetus was not macrosomic by palpation. The epidural was adequate for pain relief. The risk of vacuum delivery was discussed with patient, and the patient desired to proceed with vacuum delivery, understanding that there was a risk of fetal cephalohematoma and shoulder dystocia.
Procedure
The patient's bladder was emptied with straight catheter. A Mystic vacuum device was applied over the sagittal suture, 2 cm anterior to the posterior fontanelle. Vacuum pressure was created with hand pump to 500 mm Hg. The edge of the vacuum cup was examined, and no maternal tissue was under the cup. With left hand applying counter pressure on the vacuum cup to prevent detachment, right hand applied gentle horizontal traction along the pelvic axis, in coordination with uterine contraction and maternal pushing. Progressive descent was noted with each pull. The handle of vacuum device was gradually elevated when the perineum began to bulge. The cup was removed after delivery of the head. Mouth and nose of the infant were suctioned with a bulb at the perineum. The shoulders and the were delivered without difficulty.

The placenta was delivered intact, fundal massage was performed, and oxytocin was administered IV. The cervix and vaginal wall were thoroughly examined, and a second degree posterior midline laceration was repaired. The infant was examined after delivery, and no lacerations or bruises were observed.

Postpartum Bilateral Tubal Ligation

Date of Surgery:
Pre-op Diagnosis: Multiparity and patient desire for permanent sterilization
Post-op Diagnosis: Same
Procedure: Postpartum bilateral tubal ligation by modified Pomeroy technique
Surgeon:
Assistant:
Anesthesia: General endotracheal
EBL: 50 ml
IV Fluids: 800 ml
Urine Output: 50 ml of clear urine
Complications: None
Findings: Normal uterine fundus, tubes, and ovaries
Consent: The risks, benefits, and alternatives to tubal ligation were explained to the patient. She understood that tubal ligation is form of permanent sterilization and that the risks include injury to internal organs, intra-abdominal bleeding, and failure, which may result in future pregnancy. The patient agreed to the procedure and signed the consent.

The patient was taken to the OR and spinal anesthesia was administered. The patient was placed in the dorsal supine position, and her abdomen was prepped and draped. Two Allis clamps were placed at the lateral umbilical folds, lateral traction was applied to the clamps, and an infraumbilical skin incision was made. The fascia was grasped with the Kocher clamps and opened with Mayo scissors. The peritoneum was entered sharply.

The right cornua of the uterus was exposed with two Army-Navy retractors. The right fallopian tube was identified and brought out of the incision with a Babcock clamp, and the isthmus of the fallopian tube was elevated. A 3-cm segment of fallopian tube was ligated with a 2–0 Vicryl. A window was created in the mesosalpinx and the distal and proximal end of the tube was ligated at the base of the loop. The tube was excised and sent to pathology. The right tube was returned to the abdominal cavity. The left fallopian tube was ligated in a similar fashion. The umbilical fascia was closed with a 2–0 Vicryl suture in a continuous running fashion. The skin was closed subcuticularly with 4–0 Monocryl.

The patient tolerated the procedure well. Instrument, sponge, and needle counts were correct, and the patient was taken to the recovery room in stable condition.

Laparoscopic Tubal Fulguration

Date of Surgery:
Pre-op Diagnosis: Multiparity and patient desire for permanent sterilization
Post-op Diagnosis: Same
Procedure: Laparoscopic bilateral tubal fulguration
Surgeon:
Assistant:
Anesthesia: General endotracheal
EBL: 50 ml
IV Fluids: 1000 ml
Urine Output: 50 ml clear urine
Specimen: None
Condition: Stable
Complications: None
Findings: Normal uterus, tubes, and ovaries

Consent: The risks, benefits, and alternatives to tubal fulguration were discussed with the patient and the patient understood that tubal ligation is permanent. The risks, including injury to internal organs and intraabdominal bleeding, and failure, were explained to the patient. The patient wished to proceed and signed the consent.

Procedure

The patient was taken to the operating room with pneumatic compression stocking applied to the lower extremities. General anesthesia was administered, and the patient was placed in the dorsal lithotomy position with stirrups. The patient was prepped and draped, and the bladder was emptied.

A speculum was placed in the vagina, and the anterior lip of the cervix was grasped with a single-toothed tenaculum. A uterine manipulator was introduced. Two towel clamps were applied to the periumbilical skin to elevate the abdomen, and a vertical skin incision was made in the umbilical fold. A Veress needle was introduced into the peritoneal cavity at a straight angle. A saline drop test was performed to verify intraperitoneal placement and a pneumoperitoneum was established with CO_2 to a pressure of 15 mm Hg. A 5-mm trocar was inserted into the abdomen and intraabdominal placement was confirmed with a laparoscope.

Intraabdominal survey demonstrated a normal liver, gallbladder, and spleen, and absence of visceral injury. The pelvic anatomy was normal. A 5 mm transverse incision was made on the midline, 5 cm above the pubic symphysis. A 5-mm trocar was inserted into the abdomen under direct laparoscopic visualization. The Trendelenburg position was used to move the bowel and omentum out of pelvis.

The uterus was raised from pelvis with the uterine manipulator and the isthmus of the right fallopian tube was grasped with the bipolar grasper and elevated away from surrounding structures. Fulguration was performed and bubbling at the site of coagulation was observed. The power output of the bipolar system was 25 watts in cutting mode. Two additional fulgurations of continuous areas were performed, burning a total of 3 cm of fallopian tube. The left fallopian tube was fulgurated in a similar fashion. No bleeding was observed at the fulguration sites.

The patient tolerated the procedure well and all instruments were removed from the abdomen and vagina. Counts were correct times two. The patient was taken to the recovery room in stable condition.

Dilation and Curettage

Date of Surgery:
Pre-op Diagnosis: Missed abortion at 9 weeks gestation
Post-op Diagnosis: Same
Procedure: Suction dilation and curettage
Surgeon:
Attending:
Anesthesia: General endotracheal
IV Fluids: 250 ml
EBL: 100 ml
Urine Output: 75 ml
Specimen: Product of conception
Complications: None
Findings: 10-week sized anteverted uterus and product of conception.
Condition: Stable
Procedure: The risks, benefits, and alternatives to the procedure were explained the patient, and the patient stated that she understood the procedure and signed the consent.

The patient was taken to the operating room and general anesthesia was administered, and she was placed in the dorsal lithotomy position with stirrups. An exam under anesthesia revealed a 10-week sized anteverted uterus with a closed cervix. The patients was prepared and draped.

A weighted speculum was inserted in the vagina and a single tooth-tooth tenaculum was used to grasp the anterior lip of the cervix. The uterus was sounded to 10 cm, and the cervix was dilated with Hegar dilators to size 9. An 8 mm suction curette was inserted into the uterine fundus, and suction was applied. The products of conception were evacuated with the curette rotating on the outward movement. Gentle, sharp curettage was then performed with a large curette. The suction curette was then reintroduced to clear the uterus. The tenaculum was removed from the cervix.

The patient tolerated the procedure well, and the instrument and sponge counts were correct times two. The patient was taken to the recovery room in a stable condition.

Hysteroscopy

Date of Surgery:
Pre-op Diagnosis: Abnormal uterine bleeding (AUB)
Post-op Diagnosis: AUB, endometrial polyp
Procedure: Diagnostic hysteroscopy and dilation and curettage
Surgeon:
Attending:
Anesthesia: General endotracheal
IV Fluids: 1,000 ml
Distention Media Input: 1,500 ml normal saline.
Distention Media Output: 1,400 ml normal saline. Distention media deficit: 100 ml
EBL: 50 ml
Urine Output: 50 ml
Specimen: Endometrial lining and polyp
Complications: None
Finding: One pedunculated polyp on the posterior wall, normal uterine cavity, and normal tubal ostia.
Indication and Consent: A 40 year-old G3P3002 presented with a history of heavy vaginal bleeding. The risks, benefits, and alternatives to hysteroscopy were discussed with the patient, including the risk of uterine perforation, fluid overload, and death. She stated that she desired to proceed and signed the consent.
Procedure: The patient was taken to the operating room, general anesthesia was administered, and she was placed in the dorsal lithotomy position with stirrups. Examination under anesthesia revealed a normal anteverted uterus. The patients was then prepared and draped.

A weighted speculum was placed in the vagina, and a single-tooth tenaculum was used to grasp the anterior cervix. The uterus was sounded to 8 cm. The cervical os was dilated to 5-mm with Hegar dilators. A 5-mm 30-degree hysteroscope was introduced under visualization, and the uterus was distended with normal saline. A posterior wall pedunculated polyp was observed. The hysteroscope was then withdrawn and the cervix was dilated to accommodate a large sharp curette. The uterus was curetted in a clockwise fashion until a gritty texture was felt from all aspects of uterus. A polyp forceps was used to retrieve the large polyp from the posterior uterine wall. The polyp and endometrial scrapings were sent to pathology. The tenaculum was then removed from the cervix.

The patient tolerated the procedure well, the instrument and sponge counts were correct times two, and the patient was taken to the recovery room in a stable condition.

Laparoscopic Salpingectomy for Ectopic Pregnancy

Date of Surgery:
Pre-op Diagnosis: Right tubal pregnancy
Post-op Diagnosis: Same
Procedure: Laparoscopic left salpingectomy
Surgeon:
Assistant:
Anesthesia: General endotracheal
EBL: 100 ml
IV Fluids: 1,500 ml
Urine Output: 150 ml clear urine
Specimens: Right fallopian tube with ectopic pregnancy
Condition: Stable
Complications: None
Findings: Hemoperitoneum with 500 ml of dark blood and blood clots. The uterus, left fallopian tubes, and ovaries appeared normal. The right fallopian tube was enlarged and ruptured.
Indication and Consent: The 28-year-old G1P1 at 7 weeks by last menstrual period presented with lower abdominal pain and vaginal bleeding. Serum β-hCG was 10,000. Pelvic ultrasound revealed an empty uterus with a complex mass in the right adnexa with free fluid. The patient was diagnosed with ruptured ectopic pregnancy. The risks, benefits, and alternatives of laparoscopic surgery were discussed with the patient. The patient understood the risks, including injury to bowel, bladder, ureters, future infertility, laparotomy, and death. The patient agreed to the procedure and signed the consent.
Procedure

The patient was taken to the operating room and pneumatic compression stockings were applied to her legs. General anesthesia was administered and the patient was placed in the dorsal lithotomy position with stirrups. Examination under anesthesia revealed a normal-sized, anteverted uterus and right adnexal mass. The patient was prepared, draped, a Foley catheter inserted, and the bladder was emptied.

A speculum was placed into the vagina, and the anterior lip of the cervix was grasped with a single-tooth tenaculum. A uterine manipulator was introduced, and two Alice clamps were applied to elevate the umbilicus. A 10 mm vertical skin incision was made across the umbilical folds. Two Kocher clamps were used to grasp the fascia, which was cut. The peritoneum was opened with scissors. A 10-mm balloon trocar was inserted into the abdomen, and the balloon was inflated, and the trocar was locked. Intra-abdominal placement was confirmed with the laparoscope. A pneumoperitoneum was created with CO_2 to the pressure of 15 mm Hg.

An intraabdominal survey demonstrated a hemoperitoneum. The liver, gallbladder, and spleen were normal. The right fallopian tube was severely ruptured and unrepairable. The left fallopian tube was normal. The decision was made to proceed with right salpingectomy. Two 5-mm trocars were inserted in the bilateral lower quadrants (8 cm from the midline) under direct laparoscopic visualization. Trendelenburg position was used to improve pelvic exposure.

The right fallopian tube was elevated away from the pelvic sidewall with an atraumatic grasper. The fallopian tube proximal to the implantation site was clamped, coagulated, and transected with a 5-mm PlasmaKinetic forceps. The mesosalpinx was coagulated and cut. The tube and product of gestation were freed and placed in the anterior cul-de-sac.

The 10-mm laparoscope was withdrawn and an Endo Catch pouch was introduced through the umbilical trocar and advanced to the specimen under the direct vision with the 5-mm laparoscope. The specimen was placed in the pouch and retrieved from the umbilical incision.

The abdomen and pelvis was inspected, and good hemostasis was observed at the resection site. All instruments were removed from the abdomen and vagina. The pneumoperitoneum was released, and instrument counts were correct. The umbilical fascia was closed with 2–0 Vicryl, and skin incisions were closed with subcuticular 4–0 Monocryl. The patient was taken to the recovery room in stable condition.

Total Abdominal Hysterectomy

Date of Surgery:
Pre-op Diagnosis: Uterine leiomyoma
Post-op Diagnosis: Same
Procedure: Total abdominal hysterectomy
Surgeon:
Assistant:
Attending:
Anesthesia: General endotracheal
EBL: 300 ml
IV Fluids: 1,500 ml
Urine Output: 200 ml clear urine
Specimens: Uterus
Complications: None
Finding: 10-week-sized uterus with multiple leiomyomas and normal tubes and ovaries.

Indication and Consent

The 48-year-old female, G3P3, presented with a long history of menorrhagia and uterine leiomyoma. Risks, benefits, and alternatives were discussed with the patient, including wound, infection, bowel, bladder, ureter injury, and death. The patient desired to proceed with hysterectomy and signed the consent.

Procedure

The patient was taken to the operating room and pneumatic compression stockings were applied to her legs. General anesthesia was obtained and examination under anesthesia demonstrated 10 week size uterus. The patient was prepared and draped in dorsal supine position, and a Foley catheter was inserted to empty the bladder.

A Pfannenstiel skin incision was made and the incision was carried down to the fascia with a Bovie. The fascia was incised and the incision was extended laterally. The inferior fascia was grasped with Kocher clamps, and the rectus and pyramidalis muscles were dissected off with Mayo scissors. The superior aspect of fascia was elevated with Kocher clamps, and the rectus muscle was dissected off. Hemostasis was achieved with the Bovie, and the rectus muscle was separated in the midline down to the pubic symphysis. Pre-peritoneal fatty tissue was bluntly dissected to expose the peritoneum, and the peritoneum was entered, followed by extension of the peritoneal incision superiorly and inferiorly to the bladder reflection. Intraabdominal survey revealed a uterus with multiple leiomyoma and normal tubes and ovaries.

An O'Conner-O'Sullivan retractor was placed, with the bowel packed away using moist sponges. The Long Kelly clamps were placed along the cornua of uterus. The round ligament was identified and cut with the Bovie, and the anterior broad ligament was dissected to the midline. The bladder was dissected off the lower uterine segment and cervix with Metzenbaum scissors. A window was created in the posterior leaf, and the ovarian ligament and fallopian tube were clamped, cut, and doubly ligated.

The uterine vessels were skeletonized, doubly clamped, and cut. The pedicles were suture-ligated, and the cardinal ligament and uterosacral ligament were clamped, cut, and suture-ligated. Curved Heaney clamps were placed at the angles of the vagina. The cervix was cut from the vaginal cuff with scissors. The vaginal angle was closed with a Heaney stitch and tied to the uterosacral ligament. The vaginal cuff was then closed with a continuous-running suture, with good hemostasis noted.

The pelvis was irrigated with warm normal saline. All instruments were removed from the abdomen and the counts were correct times two. The fascial layer was closed with 2–0 PDS loop. The skin was closed with a sub-cuticular 4–0 Monocryl. The patient was taken to the recovery room in a stable condition.

Total Vaginal Hysterectomy

Date of Surgery:
Pre-op Diagnosis: Menorrhagia
Post-op Diagnosis: Same
Procedure: Total vaginal hysterectomy
Surgeon:
Assistant:
Attending:
Anesthesia: General endotracheal
EBL: 100 ml
IV Fluids: 1500 ml
Urine Output: 100 ml clear urine
Specimens: Uterus
Complications: None
Findings: Normal-sized uterus with mild prolapse.
Procedure:

The risks, benefits, indication, and alternatives to transvaginal hysterectomy were reviewed with the patient, and the patient consented to the procedure and signed the consent form.

The patient was taken to the operating room and pneumatic compression stockings were applied to her legs. General anesthesia was administered, and the patient was placed in the dorsal lithotomy position. Examination under anesthesia demonstrated a normal sized uterus. The patient was prepped and draped, a Foley catheter was inserted, and the bladder was emptied.

A weighted speculum was placed in the vagina, and the anterior and posterior cervix was grasped with a double-toothed tenaculum. A circumferential incision was made with a Bovie at cervicovaginal junction to the depth of the paracervical fascia, allowing the cervix to separate from the vagina mucosa. The posterior cul-de-sac was then entered with Mayo scissors with the scissor tips oriented towards the uterus. The midline posterior peritoneum was sutured to the vaginal mucosa, the weighted speculum was removed, and a long Steiner speculum was inserted into the cul-de-sac.

The uterosacral ligaments were clamped, cut, and suture-ligated. The cardinal ligaments were clamped, cut, and suture ligated. The peritoneum was elevated and entered sharply. A right-angle retractor was inserted into the vesicouterine space, the uterine vessels were identified, clamped, and cut. The pedicles were doubly ligated. The broad and round ligaments were clamped, cut, and suture-ligated. The ovarian ligaments and fallopian tubes were clamped, cut, and doubly ligated. The uterus was removed through the vagina, and the ovaries and tubes were visibly normal. Examination of all the pedicles demonstrated good hemostasis. The vaginal angles were sutured to the uterosacral ligaments. The vaginal cuff and the posterior peritoneum were closed with figure-8 sutures.

Instruments were removed from the vagina, all counts were correct times two, and the patient was taken to the recovery room in stable condition.

Laparoscopic Assisted Vaginal Hysterectomy

Date of Surgery:
Pre-op Diagnosis: Uterine leiomyoma
Post-op Diagnosis: Same
Procedure: Laparoscopic assisted vaginal hysterectomy and bilateral salpingo-oophorectomy
Surgeon:
Assistant:
Anesthesia: General endotracheal
EBL: 100 ml
IV Fluids: 1,500 ml
Urine Output: 200 ml clear urine
Specimens: Uterus, tubes, and ovaries
Complications: None
Findings: Uterus with multiple leiomyomas. Normal Fallopian tubes and ovaries.
Procedure:

The risks, benefits, and alternatives of the procedure were discussed with the patient, and the patient agreed to the procedure and signed the consent.

The patient was taken to the operating room and pneumatic compression stockings were applied to her lower extremities. General anesthesia was obtained and the patient was placed in the dorsal lithotomy position with stirrups. Examination under anesthesia revealed an enlarged 12 week sized uterus. The patient was prepped and draped, a Foley catheter was inserted, and the bladder was emptied.

A speculum was placed into the vagina, and the anterior lip of the cervix was grasped with a single-toothed tenaculum. A uterine manipulator was inserted. Two towel clamps were applied to the periumbilical skin to elevate the abdomen. A 15 mm vertical skin incision was made in the umbilical fold, and a Veress needle was introduced into the peritoneal cavity at a straight angle. A saline drop test was conducted to confirm intraperitoneal placement. A pneumoperitoneum was established with CO_2 to a pressure of 15 mm Hg. A 5-mm trocar was inserted into the abdomen, and intraabdominal placement was verified visually with a laparoscope.

Intraabdominal survey demonstrated a normal liver, gallbladder, and spleen. An enlarged uterus with normal ovaries and tubes was observed. Two 5-mm trocars were inserted in the lower quadrants 8 cm from the midline under laparoscopic visualization.

The uterus was elevated from the pelvis with a uterine manipulator, and the right ovary was retracted anteriorly with an atraumatic grasper. The IP ligament was clamped, coagulated, and transected with a 5-mm LigaSure device. Peristalsis of the right ureter was noted at the pelvic brim. The round and broad ligaments were transected with a LigaSure device. The procedure was repeated on the left side, and the pneumoperitoneum was released.

The patient was repositioned in dorsal lithotomy position. The cervix was grasped with a double-toothed tenaculum, and a circumferential incision around the cervix was made with a Bovie. The posterior cul-de-sac was entered sharply with Mayo scissors. Significant uterine descent was noted after the uterosacral and cardinal ligaments were sequentially clamped, transected, and suture-ligated. The anterior cul-de-sac was then entered, and the uterine vessels were identified, clamped, cut, and ligated. The uterus, tubes, and ovaries were delivered intact through the vagina.

The vaginal angles were transfixed to the uterosacral ligaments, and the vaginal cuff was closed with the figure-8 sutures. The pneumoperitoneum was reestablished, the pelvis was inspected, and no active bleeding was visible. All instruments were removed from the abdomen and vagina, counts were correct times two, and the patient was taken to the recovery room in stable condition.

Total Laparoscopic Hysterectomy

Date of Surgery:
Pre-op Diagnosis: Uterine leiomyoma
Post-op Diagnosis: Same
Procedure: Total laparoscopic hysterectomy and bilateral salpingo-oophorectomy
Surgeon:
Assistant:
Attending:
Anesthesia: General endotracheal
EBL: 250 ml
IV Fluids: 2000 ml
Urine output: 150 ml clear urine at the end of the procedure
Specimen: Uterus, tubes, and ovaries
Complications: None
Findings: Enlarged uterus with multiple leiomyomas. Normal tubes and ovaries.
Procedure

The risks, benefits, indication, and alternatives of laparoscopic hysterectomy were reviewed with the patient, and the patient agreed to the procedure and signed the consent form. The patient was taken to the operating room and pneumatic compression stockings were applied to the lower extremities, general anesthesia was administered, and the patient was placed in the dorsal lithotomy position. Examination under anesthesia demonstrated an enlarged uterus. The patient was prepped and draped, and a Foley catheter was inserted. A uterine manipulator with colpotomy ring was attached to the cervix at cervicovaginal reflection, and the occluder balloon was inflated.

Two Alice clamps were applied to the lateral umbilical folds, a vertical skin incision was made across the umbilical folds, and the fascia was grasped with 2 Kocher clamps and cut. Two stay-sutures were placed on the fascia, and the peritoneum was opened with scissors. A 10-mm Hasson trocar was inserted into the abdomen, and intraabdominal placement of the trocar was verified laparoscopically. The trocar was sutured to the fascia. A pneumoperitoneum was created with CO_2 to a pressure of 15 mm Hg.

An intraabdominal survey demonstrated a normal liver, gallbladder, and spleen. An enlarged uterus and normal tubes and ovaries were noted. Two 5-mm trocars were inserted in the lower quadrants, two fingerbreadths from the anterior-superior iliac spines. A 5-mm trocar was inserted in the midline between the pubic symphysis and umbilicus. Trendelenburg was used to increase pelvic exposure.

The uterine cornua was grasped with an atraumatic grasper, and the uterus was retracted. The peritoneum lateral to the infundibulopelvic ligament was opened with monopolar scissors. A window was created beneath the IP ligament. The ureter was visualized with peristalsis. The IP ligament was clamped, coagulated, and transected with the PlasmaKinetic forceps, and the round and broad ligaments were clamped and cut. The vesicouterine peritoneum was opened with monopolar scissors, and the bladder was dissected off the lower uterine segment and upper vagina. The uterine vessels were identified along the uterus, and the PK forceps were used to coagulate and cut the uterine vessels.

The vagina was incised circumferentially along the cervicovaginal junction. The uterosacral and cardinal ligaments and vagina were detached from the cervix. The pneumo-occluder balloon was deflated, and the uterus, tubes, and ovaries were removed through the vagina. The vaginal cuff was closed laparoscopically with Vicryl suture in a continuously running fashion. The suture was anchored with a Laparo-Tie at both ends. The pelvis was irrigated with normal saline, and good hemostasis was visualized.

All instruments were removed from the abdomen, and the fascia at the umbilicus was closed with Vicryl suture. The skin incisions were closed in a subcuticular fashion. Counts were correct times two, and the patient was taken to the recovery room in stable condition.

Labor and Delivery Notes and Orders

History and Physical Examination

Date and Time:
Last menstrual period 01/10/13, consistent with an EDC 10/17/13
Ultrasound 05/15/13 (18 wks), consistent with an EDC 10/20/13
Clinical EDC: 10/17/13
Chief Complaint: Contractions and SROM at 1200
HPI: 24 year old G2P1001 at 38 weeks by last menstrual period is consistent with ultrasound at 18 weeks has had contractions with leaking of fluid from vagina at 1200. Contractions are now regular and occur every 5 minutes. She has felt fetal movements and denies having vaginal bleeding.
Prenatal Care: Starting at 14 wks
Past Obstetric History
  NSVD at 39 weeks, male, 7 pounds and 3 oz
  Present pregnancy
Past Gynecologic History: No abnormal Pap smears. Positive Chlamydia in 2012 was treated with doxycycline and ceftriaxone.
PMH: No diabetes mellitus, hypertension, asthma, or thyroid disease
Surgical History: None
Family History: Mother with hypertension, no history of birth defects
Social History: No tobacco, alcohol or drug abuse, married
Meds: Prenatal vitamins
Allergies: NKDA
Prenatal Laboratory Studies:
Physical Examination
Vital Signs: BP 115/62, P 80, R 18, T 37.5
Heart: RRR
Lungs: Clear to auscultation
Abd: Nontender, gravid
Ext: Trace edema in bilateral extremities, DTRs 2+
Sterile Speculum Examination: positive vaginal pooling, positive ferning
Sterile Vaginal Examination: 3 cm/80%/–3/mid/soft cervix
FHT: 120s. Moderate variability, 15 for 15 accelerations, no decelerations
TOCO: Contractions every 6 minutes
Ultrasound: cephalic, anterior placenta, amniotic fluid index 5.0 cm, EFW 4300 gm
Assessment
  1. 24 year old G2P1001 at 38 wks by last menstrual period consistent with an ultrasound at 18 weeks
  2. Early labor: status/post SROM, inactive labor, fetal heart tracing
Plan
  3. CEFM with tocodynamometry
  4. Labor augmentation with oxytocin.

Admission Orders

1. **Admit to** labor and delivery
2. **IV** NS at 100 ml/hr
3. Sips of water and ice chips
4. CBC, type and screen

5. If no prenatal care, order prenatal labs including rapid HIV, UA and culture, and gonococcus/Chlamydia. Group B streptococcus culture and urine drug screen as indicated.

6. **Pain Management**
   Butorphanol (Stadol) 1–2 mg IV.
   Epidural when patient requests

5. **Magnesium Sulfate for preterm labor or Preeclampsia**
4–5 g bolus, then 2g IV/hr. Continue postpartum 20 g/500 ml LR at 2g/hr IV for 24 hr.

6. **Labor Induction and Augmentation**
Oxytocin 1–2 mU/min, increase by 2 mU/min every 15 min to maximum 32 mU/min.
Cervix ripening with misoprostol (Cytotec) 25 mcg per vagina q4–6h

7. **Postpartum Hemorrhage**
Oxytocin 20–40 units IV
Methergine 0.2 mg IM
Carboprost (Hemabate) 0.25 mg IM
Misoprostol (Cytotec) 1,000 mcg per rectum

8. **Antibiotics**
Group B streptococcus prophylaxis: penicillin 5 million units IV then 2.5–3 million units IV q4h.
Chorioamnionitis: ampicillin 2 g q6h and gentamicin 1.5 mg/kg q8h (use clindamycin instead of ampicillin if allergic to β-lactam). If cesarean is performed, add Metronidazole (Flagyl) 500 mg q12h
Endometritis: clindamycin 900 mg q8h and gentamicin 5.1 mg/kg once a day

Normal Vaginal Delivery Note

20 year old G2 P2 delivered vaginally under epidural anesthesia. Infant was suctioned with bulb syringe on the perineum. The cord was clamped and cut. Placenta was delivered intact with normal 3-vessel cord.

The fundus was firm after fundal massage and IV Pitocin. No cervical, vaginal, or perineal lacerations were visible. Male infant weighs 3,500 grams, and Apgar score was 8 at 1 min and 9 at 5 min. Estimated blood loss was 250 ml.

Postpartum Note

Subjective:
· Describe the amount of lochia, voiding, walking, flatus, bowel movement, nausea and vomiting, and breastfeeding.
· If preeclamptic: headaches, scotomata, and RUQ pain
· Lightheadedness, dyspnea
Objective:
· Vital signs — temperature and Tmax, P, RR, blood pressure, I/O's
· Lungs — Clear to auscultation
· Cardiovascular — RRR with II/VI SEM
· ABD — Fundus location, firm, tender, include dressing and incision (dressing is usually removed on post op day #2)
· Extremities — edema, calf pain
· Breast and perineum exams if indicated
· Laboratory results
Assessment:
· Status/post SVD — doing well.
· Postpartum day or Postoperative day #_____

· Labs, chest X-ray.
· Birth control method:
· Breastfeeding or bottle feeding
· Pregnancy induced hypertension — blood pressure stable.
· Postpartum Hemorrhage —. Hemoglobin and hematocrit _____. Symptoms.
· Anemia: symptoms.
Plan:
· Routine postpartum care
· Anemia: ferrous sulfate 325 mg tid po

Discharge Note

Normal Vaginal Delivery
Routine postpartum patients can be discharged 24–48 hours after delivery.
Most patients go home on postpartum day #1. Infants should be hospitalized
for a minimum of 24 hours.

Cesarean Section
1. Cesarean-section patients can be discharged 3 days post-op on postoperative day #3.
2. Remove dressing on POD #2.
3. For Pfannenstiel incisions, remove staples on POD #3, and apply Steri-strip.
4. For vertical skin incisions, remove staples on POD #5, and apply Steri-strip.

Discharge Medications
1. Progestin-only pills, Depo Provera, NSAIDs, and narcotics
2. Iron if anemia
3. Estrogen-containing birth control pills may be started 3 weeks after delivery.

Obstetrical Discharge Dictation

Patient Name:
Medical record number:
Name and Title: _____
Date of Admission:
Date of Discharge:
Admission Diagnosis:
IUP at _____ weeks
Admission diagnosis: preterm labor, preeclampsia, or spontaneous labor
Other diagnoses:
Discharge Diagnosis:
IUP at _____ weeks, delivered
Admission diagnosis: resolved, improved, or treated
Other diagnoses:
Procedures Performed: EFM, ultrasound, cesarean section.
Complications: Bladder laceration
Consultation: Maternal fetal medicine
History of Present Illness (HPI)
Patient is ____ years old G__P___, LMP__, EDD___ by LMP consistent with
__ week ultrasound or by __ week ultrasound not consistent with LMP, presented to _____ hospital with complaint of _____. Describe presentation of the
illness.
Prenatal Laboratory Studies:

Past OB History
Year of delivery, vaginal or cesarean, birth weight, complication
Year of delivery, vaginal or cesarean, birth weight, complication
PMH:
PSH:
Social History: Habits
Family History: pertinent
ROS: pertinent
Problem List
1. Intrauterine pregnancy: nonstress test, ultrasound, labs
2. Primary diagnoses
3. Other diagnosis:
Disposition
1. Discharge: home
2. Follow-up appointment: where, when
3. Instructions: activity, diet, and precautions
4. Discharge medications: name, dose, frequency, and route

Index